Keto Diet

© **Copyright 2021 - All rights reserved.**

This document is geared towards providing exact and reliable information in regards to the topic and issue covered. The publication is sold with the idea that the publisher is not required to render accounting, officially permitted, or otherwise, qualified services. If advice is necessary, legal or professional, a practiced individual in the profession should be ordered.

- From a Declaration of Principles which was accepted and approved equally by a Committee of the American Bar Association and a Committee of Publishers and Associations.

In no way is it legal to reproduce, duplicate, or transmit any part of this document in either electronic means or in printed format. Recording of this publication is strictly prohibited and any storage of this document is not allowed unless with written permission from the publisher. All rights reserved.

The information provided herein is stated to be truthful and consistent, in that any liability, in terms of inattention or otherwise, by any usage or abuse of any policies, processes, or directions contained within is the solitary and utter responsibility of the recipient reader. Under no circumstances will any legal responsibility or blame be held against the publisher for any reparation, damages, or monetary loss due to the information herein, either directly or indirectly.

Respective authors own all copyrights not held by the publisher.

The information herein is offered for informational purposes solely, and is universal as so. The presentation of the information is without contract or any type of guarantee assurance.

The trademarks that are used are without any consent, and the publication of the trademark is without permission or backing by the trademark owner. All trademarks and brands within this book are for clarifying purposes only and are the owned by the owners themselves, not affiliated with this document.

Table of Contents

Introduction 1

Chapter One: Ketogenic Diet Basics 3

Chapter Two: Understanding the Keto Diet 33

Chapter Three: Benefits of Keto Diet 37

Chapter Four: Basics of Planning Meals 45

Chapter Five: Setting up a Plan 65

Conclusion 101

Preview Of Intermittent fasting: Beginners Guide To Weight Loss For Men And Women With Intermittent Fasting 103

Introduction

The Keto Diet is the new trend in smart eating to lose weight – the reason why it has been able to capture such attention is because of its unique approach. The Keto Diet is all about eating high contents of fat and low contents of carb. When people first hear this they're always surprised because how can eating more fat make us slimmer? Well, that's because fats have been heavily stigmatized which is why all of us believe that it's only fats that make us fat when actually it's the carbs and sugars that we consume every day.

There are fats that are terrible for your body and you should avoid them, but there are also some good fats that help your body to absorb more vitamins and minerals from the food you consume. A high-fat diet doesn't just help you to lose weight, but also improves your cognitive abilities, cholesterol and even provides safety against many diseases.

The purpose of a keto is to make your eating habits a little more natural so that you stop consuming food that is artificial and fattening and instead consume food that is full of fats such as butter, cheese, nuts and fish.

In this book, you will learn everything about the keto diet – what it is all about, how it works, what are the benefits, how to follow it and how to keep yourself motivated.

Thanks again for purchasing this book, I hope you enjoy it!

Chapter One:
Ketogenic Diet Basics

Ketogenic diet is a diet that places and trains your body to be in a state wherein it primarily uses fat for energy. It achieves this through a natural metabolic process of your body called Ketosis that uses fat to create fuel for your body. A ketogenic diet has many similarities to the Atkins diet and many other low-carb diets. It has been known by several different names like low carb high fat, low carb diet and of course, the ketogenic diet.

The ketogenic diet can be implemented by discarding most of the sugars and starches in your diet and by eating healthy fats, moderate amounts of protein and very low carbs. With little carbohydrates in your diet, your body does not receive enough glucose to keep up with your body's caloric requirements. This eventually results in decreasing blood sugar levels in your body as it uses up glucose for its functions. When you eat foods that are high in carbs, your body automatically produces insulin and glucose. Insulin is made to process the glucose that is in your bloodstream by moving it around the body. Glucose is easy for your body to convert and be used for energy. Therefore, it gets chosen over all other energy sources.

As blood sugar level decreases, it looks for the stored glycogen present in your body and breaks it down to glucose and dissolves it in your blood to be distributed throughout your body. However, glycogen stores would also eventually run out. And when it does, your body would start to use fats as a source of energy for functions in its different parts and produce ketones when the liver processes it. Since glucose is used as the primary energy source, the fat in your body isn't needed and gets stored. With a normal, high carb diet, your body uses glucose as its main form of energy. By lowering the carb intake, the body is put into ketosis. These fats could come from the food that you eat, from your meals or from the fat that your body stores. This is what is called ketosis.

When you hit ketosis, your body starts being very efficient at burning fat to create energy. It turns fat in the liver into ketones that supply energy to the brain. Many studies have shown that a keto diet can help you to improve your health and lose some weight. It can also help with Alzheimer's disease, epilepsy, cancer and diabetes.

The primary advantage of following a ketogenic diet is that it restores the capability of your body to use both fat and glucose as fuel to meet its energy or caloric needs. Your body is designed to use both glucose and fat as fuel. However, due to eating a high carbohydrate diet for most of their lives, many people lack the ability to use fat for the body's energy needs. This results in bodies that have a hard time maintaining a healthy weight and a healthy body fat percentage, both of which contribute to poor health. In fact, even if you are not overweight or obese, you may still have excess visceral fat, which is wrapped around your organs like your liver, pancreas and kidneys.

With a ketogenic diet, your body restores its flexibility to use both glucose and fat as fuel for its energy needs. This flexibility keeps your fat cells, both visceral and subcutaneous (the fat located under your skin and on top of your muscles), in check by using the stored energy found in those fat cells. This would, in turn, reduce the risks of having diseases involved with having high-fat stores, specifically visceral fat:

- Type 2 Diabetes
- Coronary Artery/ Heart Disease

- Colorectal Cancer
- Breast Cancer
- High Cholesterol
- High Blood Pressure
- Metabolic Syndrome
- Alzheimer's Disease
- Stroke
- Dementia

Other than decreasing risks of said diseases, this flexibility contributes to losing excess fat and weight in a manageable manner. Normally, while and after losing some weight, your body would feel less sated after eating the same meal you ate before the weight loss process started.

And in addition to this, you might feel an increase in appetite to compensate especially if you've been depriving yourself. However, when your body is in a state of ketosis, ketones help your body manage the hormones that decrease your satiety after meals and increase your appetite and hunger. With this, you lose weight without fighting your body to gain it back through its natural responses as to what it believes to be starvation.

Moreover, being able to utilize glucose and fat for energy prevents you from experiencing the big swings that affect your mental focus, making you hungry and irritable. When glucose runs out, ketones are readily available to fuel your brain. Even better, ketones give your brain a boost, enabling you to have better focus and concentration.

Lastly, the ketogenic diet has long been used for therapy of epilepsy. This diet has been recommended for children with uncontrolled epilepsy since the 1920's. It only disappeared from popular practice when the anti-seizure medication was made available. However, unlike the anti-seizure medicine currently available, the ketogenic diet does not cause extreme side effects on patients; like drowsiness, reduced concentration, personality changes and reduced brain function.

Starting Information & Tips

The Standard Ketogenic Diet (SKD) means that 70 percent of your diet should be in the form of healthy fats, 25 percent in the form of protein and 5 percent of carbohydrates. The percentages would be based on your daily caloric requirement that is unique for every person. Since you may need to increase your caloric intake due to higher needs, you may increase the percentage of healthy fats in your diet and your body can still achieve ketosis.

Other variations of the ketogenic diet that are tweaked based on certain needs are listed down below:

Targeted Ketogenic Diet (TKD)

This type of ketogenic diet is recommended for those who engage in physical fitness. In TKD, 30 to 60 minutes before exercise, you would eat the entirety of your carbohydrates for the day in one meal. The idea of this approach is to use the energy provided in this carbohydrate meal for your fitness activities before it disrupts your body's state of ketosis.

Cyclic Ketogenic Diet (CKD)

This approach is intended for people who have a high rate of physical activities like athletes and bodybuilders. When following CKD, you switch between a ketogenic diet, and after that you follow it with a few days of high carbohydrate consumption (9 to 12 times the carbohydrates in SKD), more commonly called, "carb loading." This approach takes advantage of the body's response to high blood sugar levels from a high carbohydrate diet, which is to store it in the body's muscles and fat cells. Having this abundance of stored energy and the body able to utilize both glucose and fat for energy, it can use this energy to keep the body going during high rates of physical activity.

High-Protein Ketogenic Diet

This is a method used to ease into a Standard Ketogenic Diet when the weight is beyond the normal levels. In this approach, your protein consumption in an SKD is increased by 10 percent and your fat consumption is reduced by 10 percent. This helps those with obesity to help suppress their appetite and reduce their food intake.

Restricted Ketogenic Diet:

This method was successfully used for a brain tumor patient. In this approach, carbohydrate and calorie intake are restricted for your body to deplete glycogen stores and to start producing ketones. Since cancer cells can only feed on glucose, they are starved to death while your body thrives on ketones. It starts with a water fasting regimen and proceeds to only have a Ketogenic Diet of 600 calories a day. After two months, ketosis is in full effect and no discernable brain tumor tissue can be detected.

Only the high protein ketogenic and the standard diets have had extensive studies done on them. The targeted and cyclical diets are more advanced and are only used by athletes and bodybuilders. Even though there are several different types of this diet, the standard ketogenic diet has been researched the most and is, therefore, the one that is usually recommended.

The reason why ketogenic diets are effective lies in the functional property of fat adaption. Your body needs to be told that it has to derive its energy from fats. The biggest challenge in this regard is to keep the body programmed to this state, on a regular basis. In order to maintain ketosis, here are a few tips that you must pay heed to.

Tip 1: Drink Enough Water

You must drink a healthy amount of water to maintain a healthy body. This is a fact that all of us know and are told about time and again. However, it has also proven to be the most difficult advice to follow. The modern lifestyle is so consuming that we mostly forget simple things like keeping our bodies hydrated and eating our meals on time. It is a good idea to drink around 4 glasses of water, first thing in the morning and another 4 glasses of water before the clock strikes noon.

Tip 2: Fast Once In A While

Like we said, our bodies fail to use up the fat stores because we never, ever fast. The body is pre-programmed to run ketosis as and when the body starves. Therefore, if you are finding it hard to get your body into ketosis or maintain the ketosis state of the body, you can fast intermittently. Fasting also helps in reducing food intake and manages appetites and cravings, both of which are crucial for your diet plan. However, be sure to go on a low-carb diet for a few days before fasting intermittently. The sudden lack of sugar in the body may land you up in a hypoglycemic state.

A daylong fast can be easily broken down into two phases. The first phase extends from the first meal you consume to the last meal you eat for the day. This is the build-up phase. The second phase, which extends from your last meal for the day to the first meal of the next day, is the cleansing phase. Ideally, the cleansing phase must be longer than the build-up phase. Whenever you fast, be sure to keep your body hydrated and eat good fats like butter and coconut oil. These additions play an instrumental role in boosting up the ketone production of the body and help to maintain a healthy insulin level.

Tip 3: Add Good Salts

The high insulin levels of the body, when it is in glycolysis, affect the functioning of the kidney in such a manner that the body retains sodium. As a result, the sodium-potassium ratio destabilizes. This is why most people are advised to reduce their sodium intake. On the other hand, when on a ketogenic diet, the insulin levels are normal and the kidney functioning allows sodium excretion more effectively.

As a result, the body needs sodium to ensure proper functioning. Never make the mistake of avoiding salts when running your body on a ketogenic diet. There are several ways by which you can increase the sodium levels of the body. Some of the best ways include having broth, eating sprouted pumpkin seeds, eating cucumber as part of the salad for natural sodium and adding a pinch of salt to almost everything you eat.

Tip 4: Exercise

Regular exercise can play a crucial role in maintaining the ketosis state of the body and avoiding deposition of glucose in body parts. Exercise allows activation of glucose transport molecules that facilitate deposition of glucose in the muscles and liver. Exercises like the ones used for resistance training also facilitate the maintenance of normal blood sugar levels.

It is important to understand in this context that overdoing exercise can result in the release of stress hormones. This, in turn, increases sugar levels of the body and destabilizes the ketosis state of the body. Regular and 'just-enough' exercise can be a great way to keep you on track.

Tip 5: Avoid Too Much Protein

Most regular diet programs recommend higher protein intake. However, excessive protein intake can initiate what is called gluconeogenesis, which again generates glucose. If you feel that your body is no longer able to maintain the ketosis state, you must take a keen look at the number of proteins that you are consuming. You may have more success with a much lower protein intake.

Tip 6: Choose What You Eat Wisely

Although the ketogenic diet recommends a reduced carbohydrate intake, it is not a good idea to remove carbs from the diet completely. Therefore, the inclusion of starchy vegetables and citric fruit is a good idea. On an odd day when you are off-ketosis, you can consume berries and potatoes. However, when on ketosis, be sure to avoid sweet potato and berry-type fruit completely.

Tip 7: Reduce Stress

Stress is the root cause of most of the problems that your body's face. In fact, an increase in the stress hormones in the body can pull you off ketosis because it increases the sugar levels substantially. Therefore, maintaining a ketosis state can be an uphill task if you are going through stressful times in your life. Managing stress is an important facet of the ketogenic diet. Adopt strategies that keep your stress levels in check if you wish to make your ketogenic diet work. In line with this objective, having adequate amounts of daily sleep and maintaining a stable lifestyle is also essential.

Who should follow this diet?

The keto diet is known in popular discourse only for weight loss, but it's about much more. In this section, we will look at who should follow this diet -

Epileptic Patients

The ketogenic diet was originally developed in the early 1900s as a means of controlling seizures in children. Fasting was long a treatment in treating epilepsy and doctors found that a high-fat diet helped mimic the metabolic response of fasting. They began treating epileptic children by feeding them a diet in which up to 90% of the calories came from fat and found a marked reduction in the seizures. Half of the children fed a ketogenic diet had a reduced number of seizures and about one in seven had a complete elimination of seizures altogether.

Some studies suggest that the ketones created by the ketogenic diet are the reason it is successful in treating epilepsy. Others believe that the depletion of glucose is the reason for its success. Whatever the reason, it has proven to be effective when medication has not.

The ketogenic diet, especially when used to treat seizures, is very intense and highly controlled and can be difficult for children to follow. Doctors usually only recommend it after multiple rounds of medication have proven unsuccessful. However, many of the epileptic children who are put on the ketogenic diet for two years or longer experience a reduction or elimination of seizures, even after they cease eating it. It does not seem to have the same effect in treating epileptic teenagers and adults, possibly because it is so strict and difficult to follow. However, they can still be treated with it as long as they are willing to follow it exactly.

The ketogenic diet for epilepsy is stricter than the ketogenic diet that many people are adhering to boost their health. Rather than a 70% fat this one requires 90% fats. Side effects can include stunted growth, constipation, kidney stones, weight loss and weaker bones. If the side effects become too much, a less intense but possibly less-effective diet, such as modified Atkins, can be implemented instead.

When an epileptic patient is starting out on the ketogenic diet, he or she may need to spend a few days in the hospital for monitoring to see what effects the diet is having. Close medical monitoring will be required, including keeping a food diary, corresponding with a dietitian and getting tested every one to three months. Hyper-vigilance for carbs is required, as they can show up in some very unexpected places. For example, most kinds of toothpaste and mouthwashes contain carbs.

Parents who place their epileptic children on a ketogenic diet will have to make substantial lifestyle changes. They will have to be able to implement the diet in such a way that the epileptic child does not see it as "unfair". He or she may see siblings enjoying sweets and feel left out. All caregivers, including babysitters, teachers and other family members, will have to be aware of the strict diet. Relatives who may want to "spoil" the child by giving him or her treats at family reunions will have to understand how serious the diet is, as one simple misstep or "cheat" can trigger seizures. Some creative ideas for handling these difficult situations include using treats other than food, such as toys, fun outings, or television time. Before Halloween one year, one dad of an epileptic child on the ketogenic diet sent out a letter to all of the homes in his neighborhood that explained why his son couldn't have candy and included a toy to give him instead. The heartwarming letter went viral.

When a medical professional advises getting off the ketogenic diet in favor of a more traditional diet that includes more carbs and protein, the transition will need to be made gradually. Especially in children, the body has become so adjusted to the ketogenic diet that the metabolic changes can be difficult to adapt to.

Type 1 Diabetics

Unlike Type 2 diabetes, Type 1 diabetes is actually an autoimmune disease in which the immune system attacks the pancreas and destroys the beta cells that detect blood sugar and create insulin. As a result, the body's cells are unable to absorb any glucose and blood sugar can build up to dangerously high levels. Type 1 diabetics usually must administer insulin through injections and constantly monitor their blood sugar levels to make sure they are within a safe range. While many people are diagnosed with it as children, half of those diagnosed are over the age of 30.

There are many complications that people with Type 1 diabetes can experience, possibly as a result of the autoimmune dysfunction rather than insulin deficiency. High blood pressure and blood sugar levels can lead to eye damage, such as diabetic retinopathy, nerve damage, kidney damage and heart disease. The challenge in successfully responding to Type 1 diabetes is not only regulating blood sugar and insulin levels but also dealing with the autoimmune problems that can lead to further complications.

Lifestyle is the most important factor in managing Type 1 diabetes. Avoiding sugar, getting regular exercise, being
 consistent with insulin injections and being aware of the symptoms of impending problems are some of the most crucial things. Lowering blood sugar, thereby lowering the need for insulin, can be very effective at managing the disease.
The ketogenic diet can be a powerful way of lowering blood sugar in patients with Type 1 diabetes. Many find that they are able to reduce their need for insulin by up to 80% or more.

When following a ketogenic diet with Type 1 diabetes, the person must be absolutely all in. There are no cheats allowed, as just one cheat meal can put the body in a dangerous, potentially deadly state known as ketoacidosis. This occurs when ketones build up in the blood, causing it to become more acidic.

The ketones, which are naturally present on the ketogenic diet, can build up to dangerously high levels as they react with the blood sugar. Diabetics on the ketogenic diet should closely monitor their ketone and glucose levels and remain carefully under a doctor's supervision.

Type 1 diabetics may need to follow a modified version of the ketogenic diet, which is more strictly controlled but more suited to the disease.

Type 2 Diabetics

Type 2 diabetes, also known as adult diabetes, is oftentimes the result of lifestyle choices that lead to chronically high levels of blood sugar, thereby leading to insulin resistance. While Type 1 diabetes is caused by the inability of the body to create insulin, Type 2 diabetes is the result of it being unable to use insulin. Increasingly unhealthy lifestyle choices are leading to children being diagnosed with Type 2 diabetes, whereby it was previously unheard of in people under the age of 50.

Diet, exercise and close monitoring of insulin levels are key to managing Type 2 diabetes. Complete lifestyle overhauls have led some people to completely reverse the symptoms and no longer need medication. The most obvious benefit is that the lowered blood sugar leads to less dependence on insulin.

The conundrum created by applying the ketogenic diet to Type 2 diabetes is that because so many people with the disease are overweight or obese, adopting a high-fat diet seems to be counterintuitive. After all, fat is a much more concentrated source of calories than carbs or protein, so it should actually lead to weight gain and exacerbate the person's health problems. However, that is a myth based on a misunderstanding of calories and the complex chemistry involved in metabolism. The fact is that not all calories are created equal and healthy fats, as opposed to carbs, can actually decrease your appetite so that you end up consuming fewer calories. Additionally, the decreased production of ghrelin, the hunger hormone and the increased production of leptin and amylin, the satiety hormones, generated by the state of ketosis further restrict the calorie intake.

As with Type 1 diabetes, people with Type 2 diabetes are at risk of developing ketoacidosis, so constant monitoring of blood sugar and ketones is important. Additionally, the ketogenic diet should be followed under a doctor's supervision.

Early-Stage Alzheimer's Patients

One of the biggest health concerns today is the risk of developing Alzheimer's disease. Alzheimer's seems to have a bit of a genetic component and is also linked with lifestyle factors. As previously mentioned, some researchers have come to call it Type 3 Diabetes because of its connection with insulin resistance and a buildup of glucose in the brain.

Preliminary studies, both in animal and human trials, indicate that the ketogenic diet is effective at restoring normal brain metabolism in people with early-stage Alzheimer's disease. It reduces and can even eliminate the buildup of unabsorbed glucose that leads to cell death while providing the brain with the superior energy provided by ketones. Ketones are able to provide all of the nutrients necessary for optimal brain function. At optimal levels they do not build up in the bloodstream, leading to the creation of the dangerous plaques and tangles that cause neurodegeneration.

As yet, there is no indication that the ketogenic diet can reverse Alzheimer's disease once it has begun. However, results so far are promising. Research over the past few decades has revealed that the brain has a high level of plasticity, meaning that neurons are able to regenerate, grow and adapt to changing needs. Ketones may be able to tap into this plasticity to help halt Alzheimer's in its tracks and future research into treatment for Alzheimer's will focus heavily on ketones.

People who are diagnosed with Alzheimer's disease tend to be older, usually over the age of 60, so implementing the changes required by the ketogenic diet can be difficult. Additionally, maintaining the person's lifestyle as much as possible is seen as a cornerstone in caring for someone with Alzheimer's, as consistency and normalcy can help deal with the emotional challenges that people with the disease face. Getting Alzheimer's patients to establish a ketogenic diet can be very difficult and will require the complete commitment of all caregivers.

People, who are at risk of developing Alzheimer's disease, because of preexisting insulin resistance, genetic factors, or environmental factors, may benefit from the ketogenic diet. It may prevent the brain decay that is characteristic of the disease.

Parkinson's Patients

Parkinson's disease is a neurodegenerative disorder caused by abnormal levels of the hormone dopamine. The dopamine-creating neurons die and the loss of dopamine results in the characteristic tremors that people with

Parkinson's experience. Additionally, they deal with problems such as depression, lack of clarity, forgetfulness and loss of physical function. The disease is progressive, so it gets worse over time. Medications are available to help manage the symptoms, but there is no cure.

Dysfunction in the mitochondria is believed to be a cause of the death of the dopamine-creating neurons, which leads to Parkinson's. The previous chapter already discussed the role of ketones in protecting and enhancing the mitochondria, so from this perspective, ketones may play a role in helping to treat Parkinson's patients. Preliminary studies in animals have shown that the ketogenic diet can improve mitochondrial function. In humans, a preliminary study has shown that one month on the ketogenic diet leads to decreased tremors, elevated mood, improved gait and increased energy.

People who are diagnosed with Parkinson's disease tend to be older, so implementing the intense lifestyle changes required by the ketogenic diet can be quite difficult. Those who participated in the preliminary testing had trouble staying on it and several quit, despite the potential for treatment. A gradual transition to the ketogenic diet may be helpful in maintaining it.

Cancer Patients

In addition to finding new medications that can potentially help cancer patients, much cancer research is now looking into the effects of diet and lifestyle as supplements to traditional treatments. Vegetable juicing and eating an organic-only diet has helped many cancer patients recover. New research is focusing on the potential of a ketogenic diet in helping to cure cancer.

One way that a ketogenic diet may benefit cancer patients is that sugar is all but eliminated. Sugar is basically what cancer cells thrive on; there is a direct correlation between sugar consumption and growth of tumors. By switching the body's energy source from glucose to ketones, the tumors become starved and may shrink.

Additionally, the benefits for mitochondrial metabolism may improve the responses of healthy cells and generate apoptosis, the body's method of intentionally destroying cancerous cells. Studies are showing that a ketogenic diet increases the oxidative stress on the mitochondria in cancer cells, making them more sensitive to chemotherapy and other traditional treatments.

Meanwhile, the mitochondria of the healthy cells are enhanced, making them less prone to the harmful effects of treatments. Cancer patients who want to adopt a ketogenic diet should consult with an oncologist who specializes in how a ketogenic diet can help with that particular type of cancer.

PCOS Patients

Polycystic ovarian syndrome, or PCOS, is a metabolic dysfunction that is closely correlated with insulin resistance. It leads to problems such as infertility, acne, dysmenorrhea (heavy periods that have intense cramping), amenorrhea (lack of periods) and hirsutism (irregular hair growth across the body). While the ovaries usually release an egg every 28 days, in women with PCOS, the eggs remain in the ovaries and turn into cysts. Over time, the cysts build up in both ovaries until there are dozens or even hundreds. Many women with PCOS treat their symptoms with medication, but the disease can also be managed and sometimes even reversed through diet.

Consistently high levels of blood sugar cause insulin resistance. The first step to treating PCOS through diet is by eliminating sugar, then reducing and eliminating all other carbs, as well. PCOS is also strongly correlated with obesity; some women develop PCOS and become obese because of the intense hormonal disruptions, while some obese women are more prone to developing PCOS. Another step towards treating the disease with diet is to lose weight. Because the weight gain tends to be at least partly hormonal, balancing the hormones is crucial.

The ketogenic diet can help women with PCOS to both balance their hormones and lose weight. Although clinical studies are few and small, case studies and anecdotal evidence regarding the success of low-carb diets in treating PCOS are impressive; the lowered insulin levels help to reverse insulin resistance and stabilize other hormone imbalances. It is not uncommon for women with PCOS who are on a low-carb diet to lose weight, achieve normal periods and even regain their fertility.

While there is little research as to the ketogenic diet specifically with women who have PCOS, preliminary results are promising. There are several foods on the ketogenic diet, such as fatty fish and nuts that are particularly helpful for those with the disease. If you have PCOS and want to try the ketogenic diet to see if it can help relieve your symptoms and even reverse the disease, talk with your endocrinologist about how it may benefit you.

People with Autism

Autism is a neurological disorder that has been on the rise, particularly in the United States. Its characteristic feature is impaired social interaction and cognitive development, including language development. The increased prevalence of autistic diagnoses has led many parents to be concerned about possible causes of autism. Some have even shunned life-saving vaccines because they are concerned that they may cause autism. Its causes seem to be varied and include genetic and environmental factors.

Treatment usually focuses on managing behavior with intense therapy; there is no known cure for autism. It is a lifelong condition and many adults with autism must either be cared for full time by a family member or live in a care home. The success of the ketogenic diet in treating neurological disorders has led to speculation about whether it may be able to benefit people with autism. Many diets have been applied to clinical studies for children with autism spectrum disorders, but the benefits seem to be minimal. However, the ketogenic diet seems to hold great promise and has already proven to help autistic children in some clinical trials.

It is not uncommon for people with autism to also suffer from seizures. The benefits of the ketogenic diet in treating seizures were described in the first section; someone with autism who also has seizures may experience diminished epileptic activity as a result of the ketogenic diet.

Autism spectrum disorders tend to display certain behaviors, including repetitive behaviors known as stimming and agitation. Mice with characteristics that mimic autism, such as repetitive behaviors and lack of social interaction, who were fed a ketogenic diet experienced reversals of the symptoms and behaved like normal mice. In clinical trials, autistic children fed a ketogenic diet experienced marked improvement in these behaviors and even showed an increase in social activity.
Autism also tends to have an effect on cognition. While some forms of autism, such as Asperger's syndrome, can lead to increased mental acuity, there is oftentimes a lack of executive function, which inhibits the person's ability to make connections between ideas. The ketogenic diet has been shown to help people with autism improve their cognitive process. This

may be because it promotes the neurotransmitter adenosine, which promotes sleep and reduces anxious behavior.

People with Mood Disorders and Mental Illness

The typical Western diet, which is high in processed foods, sugars and other carbs, triggers biological processes that induce mood disorders like depression and anxiety. Sugar is possibly the most addictive substance on the planet, so it is little wonder that it would cause problems with mood. Many people rely on antidepressants and other medications to deal with their mood disorders; however, they can also be treated naturally. Eliminating sugar is the first step. Following a ketogenic diet can dramatically improve mood.

Additionally, the neurological processes stimulated by a ketogenic diet can treat more severe mental illnesses, such as bipolar and schizophrenia. While going keto is unlikely to cure the disease, it can help to manage symptoms.

It is important to remember that mood disorders and mental illnesses are multifaceted and can be triggered by stressful events and other environmental factors; they also seem to have a genetic link. While improving the brain's chemistry, a ketogenic diet is unable to resolve these other factors that contribute to mental illness and mood disorders.

Depression:
As opposed to sadness, which is a normal emotion that everyone experiences; depression is a clinical condition in which a lowered mood persists for weeks, months and even years. It results in a severely lowered quality of life both for the depressed individual and his or her family.

Numerous case studies exist to support the idea that a ketogenic diet can help treat depression and these case studies seem to be backed by scientific evidence and data. One cause of depression is neurotoxicity spurred by imbalances of the neurotransmitters GABA and glutamate. The use of ketones is able to improve the balance, thereby alleviating some of the chemical causes of depression.

Additionally, depression and inflammation are strongly linked. Conditions such as leaky gut syndrome, which is becoming more prevalent among Westerners eating a high-carb diet, decimate the microbiome of the gut, which is responsible for much of the hormones that the body produces. This alone can lead to the chemical imbalances that are associated with depression. Leaky gut syndrome and a less-than-optimal microbiome also contribute to inflammation, which can also cause or worsen depression. The ketogenic diet eliminates the foods that lead to intestinal problems, making it ideal to treat some of the causes of depression.

Adapting a ketogenic diet is just one aspect of overcoming depression and it is not a substitute for counseling.

Anxiety:

While some stress is beneficial and necessary for daily function, anxiety refers to a large amount of stress that hampers a person to complete the tasks he or she needs to do and lowers the overall quality of life. The build-up of stress hormones, such as cortisol and adrenaline, can cause stressful events to affect a person's metabolic processes. In addition to depression, anxiety-related disorders are on the rise, especially in children, who are constantly expected to achieve increasingly high expectations. The high-sugar diet adopted by many Westerners is known to contribute to anxiety and also fuels the release of cortisol and adrenaline. Eliminating sugar and exercising regularly are important to reducing levels of stress hormones. The ketogenic diet can also help stabilize the metabolic processes that lead to anxiety and reverse the damage caused by it.

As with depression, there are numerous case studies of people who suffered from anxiety and experienced substantial relief from following a ketogenic diet. This is possible because the metabolic processes in the brain are transformed through the creation and burning of ketones for energy instead of using sugar.

Schizophrenia:

Schizophrenia is a rare but serious mental illness in which a person experiences things that are not present as if they are happening. They typically experience hallucinations, which are not limited to seeing things that are not present but can also include hearing things (the "voices" associated with schizophrenia) and feeling sensations, such as itching, that do not have a physical cause. The exact causes are not known, but there seem to be both genetic and environmental factors. Treatment for schizophrenia includes behavior modification therapy and heavy medication regimens.

People suffering from schizophrenia are at a high risk of suicide and also of harming others; many need full-time care throughout their entire lives. In laboratory trials, mice whose brains were induced to have the same chemical structure as a schizophrenic brain and who had schizophrenic behaviors were fed a ketogenic diet. After three weeks, some of their mental processes became completely normal. While there is presently no data to support the treatment of schizophrenic humans with a ketogenic diet, there is certainly promise.

Bipolar:

Bipolar is a serious mental illness in which a person swings from periods of depression to mania. Intense manic periods can cause the person to become completely detached from reality and engage in risky behaviors that he or she would not ordinarily consider. There is a high rate of suicide and other harmful behaviors associated with bipolar disorder and while some people with bipolar are able to function on their own, others need lifelong care.

Many bipolar medications are also used to treat epilepsy. Because of the ketogenic diet's success in treating epilepsy, researchers were interested to find if it could also treat bipolar. Scientific evidence says that yes, it may be able to. Seizure medications that reduce the amount of sodium in the extracellular area are the only ones that are effective at treating bipolar; the ketogenic diet is effective at achieving the same thing.

Sodium is responsible for many of the metabolic processes that occur within the brain, as keeping an optimal balance of sodium and potassium is necessary for ensuring the correct electrical function that enables communication between neurons. Whacked-out sodium levels can cause problems with the functioning of neurons, which can trigger the psychotic episodes associated with bipolar. This is the reason why bipolar medication seeks to stabilize the brain's sodium.

By helping the brain maintain optimal sodium levels, both within neurons and outside of them, the ketogenic diet is able to achieve the same effect as bipolar medication.

People with Cerebral Palsy

Cerebral palsy is a neurological condition that is usually caused by lack of oxygen during birth or during the first five years of life. The brain damage caused by the lack of oxygen can lead to problems including seizures, lack of coordination, muscle spasms, difficulty with depth perception, speech difficulties and hearing and vision problems. There is no cure for cerebral palsy, but a ketogenic diet can be part of a treatment plan to improve the quality of life for people who have it.

The ketogenic can be hugely effective at treating the seizures that are associated with cerebral palsy. Further research into how it can help other aspects of cerebral palsy, such as brain damage and muscle spasms, is necessary to see how effective it is as a global treatment.

People Who Want To Lose Weight

The body's chemistry, not the arithmetic of calories in versus calories out, is what determines whether people gain weight or lose weight. Consuming carbs leads to the production of insulin, which turns on the body's fat-producing hormones. Research is increasingly finding that insulin is directly related to weight gain. Unless you immediately burn off the sugars that you consume, they will be stored as fat. This occurs regardless of whether you are eating "diet" foods or not. The key to losing weight is not in restricting calories but in lowering your insulin levels.

People on the ketogenic diet often find that they lose weight without having to restrict calories. They feel less hungry, have a much more stable appetite and feel more satisfied after eating. Without sugar being used as the body's primary fuel source, they immediately begin to burn through fat.

Some doctors have suggested that people on the ketogenic diet immediately begin to lose water weight rather than actual fat. However, this claim comes back to the faulty reasoning about the body needing carbs for energy in the form of glucose. The ketogenic diet leads the body to respond as if it is in a state of fasting by burning through fat at a high rate.

People with Fatty Liver Disease

The liver is an organ that is part of the digestive system; it filters out toxins, synthesizes enzymes and other chemicals necessary for digestion, breaks down carbs and even helps with blood clotting! It is a very important organ and keeping it healthy is of the utmost importance. Fatty liver disease is the first in a progression of liver problems. One type is caused by alcohol consumption and the other type is correlated with genetics, obesity, cholesterol and consumption of carbohydrates. Symptoms include fatigue, weight loss, nausea, confusion, lack of clarity and overall weakness. Left untreated, it could turn into cirrhosis or scarring of the liver. Cirrhosis is a serious disease that causes fluids to accumulate throughout the body, muscles to atrophy, internal bleeding, liver failure and jaundice.

While alcohol-based fatty liver disease is treated by completely abstaining from alcohol, non-alcoholic fatty liver disease (NAFLD) can be treated through diet. Adopting a high-fat diet seems to be counter-intuitive for treating a disease characterized by the fat build-up in the liver; carbs are actually more often the culprit behind NAFLD. People with NAFLD who adopt the ketogenic diet have shown reductions in the fats in their livers and overall better liver function.

If you have NAFLD and want to get on the ketogenic diet, make sure you inform your doctor. He or she may recommend frequent testing to monitor how the diet is affecting your liver.

People with Acne

Acne is a skin condition that results from unbalanced hormones, especially insulin and cortisol. Insulin causes the creation of new skin cells and causes them to stick together, both of which can lead to breakouts. It also stimulates the production of sebum, which is a type of oil the skin produces and testosterone, which also causes acne.

Severely reducing insulin levels by following a ketogenic diet has been shown to drastically help people who suffer from acne. The thought of following a high-fat diet to decrease the skin's oil production seems counterintuitive, but again, it all comes back to the body's complex chemistry and metabolism.

Many people find that when they first begin the ketogenic diet, their acne actually gets worse. However, this is usually because hormone levels are stabilizing and inflammation is healing. A month or so in, acne begins to heal and, with time, even the scars begin to go away.

People with ADD, ADHD and Executive Dysfunctions

ADD, or attention deficit disorder and ADHD, attention deficit and hyperactive disorder, cause many children and adults to have difficulty focusing and staying on task. While some people think of the disorders as people just not being willing to sit still and be quiet, they are actually rooted in neurological processes that involve neurotransmitters and other aspects of the brain's chemistry. They are often treated with medication, although some people prefer to treat them through lifestyle and forego medication. Executive function disorders are common in people with ADD and ADHD. Think of all of the functions that an executive at an office must perform: delegate tasks to employees, manage a busy schedule, coordinate meetings, oversee various departments, etc. Imagine an office trying to function without an executive and all of the different parts are running but not being coordinated. That is what an executive function disorder looks like. People with an executive function disorder know what they need to do, but they are unable to figure out exactly how to carry out the tasks.

The ketogenic diet can be of benefit to people struggling with these disorders. Parents of children with these disorders usually restrict sugar intake, as it can lead to an increase in symptoms. Consumption of whole foods without any preservatives can help decrease symptoms, as can eating high levels of healthy fats. While there haven't been many clinical trials done regarding the benefits of the ketogenic diet for ADD, ADHD and executive function disorders, there are numerous case studies suggesting that it can be very helpful.

People with a History of Eating Disorders

Eating disorders are not primarily physical but rather psychiatric problems. They tend to have deep roots in self-image, self-esteem, self-confidence and social wellbeing. The most common eating disorder is anorexia, a condition in which sufferers have an irrational fear of weight gain and see themselves as much larger than they actually are. They starve themselves and as a result, have severe nutrient deficiencies and are severely underweight. Left untreated, anorexics can die from the disorder. People with anorexia typically have an intense fear of fat, even though carbs are much more of a culprit in terms of weight gain. Because they are in a state of starvation (as opposed to fasting), they crave sweets and may binge eat on fat-free carbs. Eating a high-fat diet is not a good idea for someone who has been struggling with anorexia.
Additionally, because it promotes weight loss, anorexics should avoid it. Another common eating disorder is bulimia, a condition in which someone binge eats and then induces either vomiting or diarrhea to rid the body of all of the calories consumed. The severe instability that the body faces can make the ketogenic diet quite dangerous. However, if done under the careful supervision of a physician and psychiatrist, people with bulimia can find that the ketogenic diet is actually very healing for both their minds and their bodies. This must be done as part of a comprehensive treatment program and not a method of losing weight (as a substitute for purging).

People with Gallbladder Problems

People with gallbladder problems or with no gallbladder should avoid the ketogenic diet because they have difficulty processing fats. The gallbladder stores bile, a chemical that helps break down fats in the intestines. With the decreased levels of bile, the fat is unable to be absorbed and a nutrient deficiency results. Additionally, the ketogenic diet can lead to gallstones, which can exacerbate existing gallbladder problems.

However, under a doctor's careful supervision, people with gallbladder issues can take some steps to enable them to follow the ketogenic diet successfully. Consuming foods that stimulate the production of bile and optimal levels of stomach acid, such as ginger, celery, cucumbers, apple cider vinegar, artichokes, asparagus and dandelion greens can help avoid some of the problems with fat absorption. Drinking plenty of water — four cups within the first hour of waking up and an additional four cups before lunch — is essential. This will mean a lot of trips to the bathroom, so you will have to decide if your lifestyle will allow you to follow the ketogenic diet with gallbladder issues.

People Who Have Had Bariatric Surgery

After having stomach-altering surgery, such as a gastric bypass, the ketogenic diet can prove to be challenging. People who have had bariatric surgery have usually struggled with morbid obesity for much of their lives and have spent just as much time trying out different diets in the attempt to lose weight. The problem is that when they are successful at losing weight, they are equally successful at gaining it back.

While the ketogenic diet provides the benefit of weight loss, it is not primarily a weight-loss tool. When people who have been on the ketogenic diet revert back to eating a moderate amount of carbs, they tend to gain back some of the weight that they lose. For someone who has had bariatric surgery, this means getting back onto the weight-loss, weight-gain roller coaster. The results can be demoralizing, especially after so much effort was put into the weight-loss surgery.

Instead, people who have had bariatric surgery are usually advised to follow a modified ketogenic diet, which allows for a high protein intake rather than a high fat intake. If you have had bariatric surgery, consult with your physician about how you can get your body into a state of ketosis without getting back onto the weight-loss, weight-gain roller coaster.

People with Kidney Problems

While the ketogenic diet is unlikely to cause harmful effects for people who don't have kidney problems, those who have pre-existing issues are more likely to experience complications. Your kidneys are the organs that filter your blood and remove toxins and other waste products to be excreted as urine. You only need one functioning kidney to live, but people who have a history of kidney problems tend to have an issue with both.

Diets that are high in protein tend to be harder on the kidneys because they cause them to work more to excrete the excess calcium, potassium, sodium and by-products of metabolizing proteins. The process of ketosis can cause kidney stones to form and also causes the blood to become more acidic, leading to potential complications for those with a kidney condition. Left untreated, kidney problems can lead to a need for dialysis, a time-consuming and taxing procedure in which the blood is artificially filtered a few times each week.

If you have pre-existing kidney problems but want to follow the ketogenic diet, consult with your doctor and only change your diet under his or her supervision. You may need to be monitored and tested frequently to ensure that the diet is not harming your kidneys.

People Who Are Underweight

While obesity is the primary factor behind many chronic diseases and is reaching epidemic proportions, there are many people who are actually underweight. This may be because of metabolic problems, such as hyperthyroidism, an intense exercise regimen, or not consuming enough calories to meet the body's nutritional needs. There could also be serious underlying health problems, especially if a person with a normal weight begins to lose weight without making any lifestyle changes. Unexpected weight loss can signal serious problems, including diabetes and cancer.

The ketogenic diet is known to induce weight loss, so even though it is much healthier than many other diets, it can have a negative effect on people who are already underweight. If you are underweight and want to begin the ketogenic diet for its health benefits, speak with your doctor. He or she may advise that you adopt a modified ketogenic diet, which will include more carbs and protein to help you gain weight while eating more foods that will induce ketosis.

People Who Should Avoid the Ketogenic Diet

If you are under any medication, breastfeeding, or have any degenerative disease, please see a doctor who understands the ketogenic diet. Your health could be aggravated due to your condition. The ketogenic diet is for the purposes of improving your health and not making things worse. It's better to be safe and consult your doctor than be sorry about it just because you failed to have a consultation.

Chapter Two:
Understanding the Keto Diet

To understand how the keto diet works, you must first know how your body converts the food that you eat into energy and how it uses it. This is done by your digestive system through digestion. Digestion is the process of breaking down food through mechanical and chemical actions. Without breaking down food into their simpler forms, your body cannot use it for energy, growth and cell repair. The food that you eat consists of nutrients that can be primarily divided into two classifications: macronutrients and micronutrients. While micronutrients help our body to repair, grow and protect itself, macronutrients provide the energy our body needs. These two nutrient subdivisions could be further divided - the macronutrients into fats, proteins and carbohydrates; and micronutrients into the vast array of vitamins and minerals.

Carbohydrates

Carbohydrates come from sugars, starches and fiber found in the fruit, grains and vegetables that you eat. These are broken down by the saliva in your mouth, small intestine and pancreas into glucose, sucrose and fructose (simple sugars). The simple sugars are for the body's immediate energy needs.

Protein

Proteins come from meat, eggs and beans that you eat. These are all broken down by the stomach, small intestines and pancreas into amino acids.

These are used by your body to create neurotransmitters, non-essential amino acids and other protein-based compounds. Excess amino acids are circulated and used to repair damaged tissues or are stored as glucose.

Fats

Fats come from oils and fat in our diet. These are broken down by the liver and pancreas into fatty acids and glycerol. These are used by the body to repair cells and make different chemicals or tissues.

Vitamins

Vitamins come from the food solids and liquid that you eat. As these are broken down by your system, the small and large intestines absorb the vitamins for use in different body functions, from fighting inflammation to repairing cell damage. These are all absorbed in the small intestines by specialized cells that pass across the intestinal lining. Your bloodstream circulates amino acids, simple sugars, glycerol and other salts and vitamins to your liver. The vessels that move white blood cells and lymph throughout the body, called as lymphatic system, circulates fatty acids and vitamins.

This whole process of digestion is controlled by your nervous system and the hormones your body produce. Your nerves cause muscles of the GI tract to contract or relax to digest food and release a substance to control the movement of food and the production of digestive juices. Your hormones, on the other hand, regulate appetite and stimulate the production of digestive juices.

There will be excess nutrients that your body won't need after this whole ordeal. Your excess blood sugar and amino acids would be stored in your body as either glycogen in liver, muscle and fat cells. The excess amino acids get stored as glucose while the excess fats get stored as triglycerides in the fat cells. Vitamins in excess are either expelled through urine, if water-soluble, or stored in the liver and fat cells, if fat-soluble.

The Fasted State

Around 2 to 8 hours after your last meal, your body enters a state of fasting. In this state, your body's blood sugar drops to a lower threshold level, which also brings down the levels of insulin in it. With the drop of glucose in your blood, a hormone from the liver, called glucagon is released to release the stored energy in your cells. This raises your glucose levels in your bloodstream, which is primarily used by the brain and red blood cells.

After these stores are used up, the body starts to be in a state of ketosis. Triglycerides are released from fat cells and are used by your muscles and liver cells as fuel. From the liver's use of triglycerides, ketones are formed and used if more energy is needed. As your body's fasted state goes further, more triglycerides are released, broken down and used for energy. As you can see, thanks to ketosis, the body can freely switch energy consumption from blood sugar to the stored glycogen, glucose and triglycerides. However, due to the high carbohydrate diets, your body had somehow gotten used to only using blood sugar for energy.

Whenever it goes down, you start getting hungry and craving for a meal with carbohydrates. If you do eat a meal without carbohydrates, you don't feel as satisfied. This does not normally occur when ketosis occurs in a fasted state due to the ketones that prevent hunger hormones from coming out and trigger hormones that signal your brain to feel sated as if you ate a meal.

Ketosis Effect

On a diet that is high or centered around carbohydrates, your body is primarily burning glucose for fuel. Since it is frequently supplied with carbohydrates through your meals, it does not adapt itself out of a glucose burning state and into fat burning. And whenever it needs more glucose, your body would just tell you that it's time to eat. As any excess in caloric intake would result in your body storing fat, it would just keep storing fat whenever you do. Since it is in a standard state of using glucose as a primary source of energy, your body won't readily use what is in its fat stores. This perpetuates a cycle of your body gaining fat from the excess caloric intake and being unable to burn it for energy.

With a ketogenic diet, the body does not primarily depend on carbohydrates for your body's daily caloric requirements. This results in your body adapting to this diet and, then naturally, switching to looking for its required energy and primarily using fat for fuel. With your body in a state of ketosis, it uses up your fat stores more readily whenever your body runs out of the fat it got from your last meal. Instead of you feeling hungry, it just uses up the stored energy in your body fat.

There are two ways that you can do for your body to achieve a state of ketosis. This is through fasting from food or substituting the carbohydrates in your diet with healthy fats, which is what the ketogenic diet does. Since fasting in the long-term is not a sustainable way to achieve ketosis, the ketogenic diet is the way to go for anyone who wants to take advantage of this fat burning state of your body. However, the ketogenic diet goes beyond the ratio of the carbohydrates, proteins and fats that are in your meals. You must eat the right nutrients to be able to healthily achieve ketosis. Doing so otherwise could lead to chronic inflammation, metabolic disorders and other degenerative diseases.

Chapter Three:
Benefits of Keto Diet

The ketogenic diet is absolutely unique and it gives you benefits that you wouldn't find in any other diet. The main aim behind the diet is to reduce your dependence on carbohydrates and inducing your body to burn more fats.

Fighting Cancer

The ketogenic diet is a natural deterrent for cancer cells. The ketogenic diet usually consists of 75 percent fat, 20 percent protein and 5 percent carbohydrates. This limits the number of carbs and sugar that you consume. Cancer cells replicate themselves throughout your body once they start growing. These cells need sugar in order to create enough energy to replicate themselves. Since the ketogenic diet eliminates intake of sugar, the cancer cells are left stranded.

The diet also reduces your intake of carbohydrates. This further helps in fighting cancer, as the cancer cells do not have an alternative source to generate energy. This does not mean that you won't have the energy that you need for daily activities. Your regular cells can use fats to generate energy but cancer cells cannot simply switch to a different source.

Helps in Weight Loss

If we consume carbohydrates, insulin is released throughout the body in order to increase blood glucose. Insulin is a type of hormone. Its basic function is to ensure that the body has enough energy for all of its needs. So, when insulin is released it further propagates the cells to save as much energy as possible. The cells initially save the energy in the form of glycogen (carbohydrates in their stored form) then later on as fat.

The ketogenic diet aims at reducing the level of carbohydrates that you consume so that they are almost negligible in your body. This prevents your body from releasing insulin. When insulin is not released in the body then there is a lack of glycogen, which the body needs in order to generate energy. Your body is forced to burn fats in order to generate energy. This helps in reducing the number of fats that are stored in your body and therefore, helps you to lose weight.

Treating Alzheimer's disease

Alzheimer is a disease that slowly deteriorates your nervous system. If it goes untreated it can even lead to Dementia. The ketogenic diet is the perfect way to treat Alzheimer's.

When you get old, the nervous system stops working properly and tends to slow down after a while. This causes mood swings, random episodes of dementia and most importantly memory loss. To prevent Alzheimer's from growing, it's important to take care of your nervous system.

The nervous system is directly linked to the brain. So, to help the brain it is important to consume healthy fats. Healthy fats make your brain more active. The ketogenic diet consists of 70 percent healthy fats and therefore it helps the brain.

Lower Blood Pressure

Elevated blood pressure can lead to many diseases including heart attack, kidney failure and others.

The ketogenic diet makes sure that you do not consume too many carbs. This reduces the blood pressure of your body. It's been seen in numerous cases that a reduction in consumption of carbs led to decreased blood pressure. The reason behind this is that a low carb diet induces the body to store fewer fluids. This includes the constituent fluids present in the blood.

A lower blood pressure reduces the risk of an early death and also makes you feel more energetic than before.

Improved brain function

The idea that the brain functions entirely on glucose is simply untrue. The brain only needs about 40 grams of glucose per day (that level may vary according to the individual), which can be synthesized from proteins through the process of gluconeogenesis. Once the body becomes fully adapted to the ketogenic diet, the brain can meet 75% of its energy needs from ketones, with the remaining 25% coming from the glucose made from proteins.

The brain actually contains astrocytes, which produce ketones. This fact indicates that the brain actually does function more optimally on ketones. Also, the fact that the ketogenic diet was originally established to treat neurological disorders, especially epilepsy, shows how important they are to establishing optimal brain function.

Ketones are actually a more efficient fuel for the brain and create fewer waste products than glucose.

Over time, the brain clears out all of the waste products generated by relying on glucose for energy. Running on ketones, it is able to establish optimal sodium levels between neurons, thereby decreasing the symptoms of diseases like depression, anxiety, schizophrenia and bipolar. Damaged neurons can begin to heal and even regenerate. Thoughts become clearer, mood increases and the brain operates optimally.

Improved nutrition

Without eating many fruit and limiting the vegetables consumed, one concern about the ketogenic diet is that over time, it can lead to nutrient deficiencies. While it may be beneficial in the short term to help achieve weight loss and other health goals, over the long term, it can be harmful because it does not provide complete nutrition. The only thing necessary to induce ketosis is very few carbs and lots of fat. This can be accomplished by drinking canola oil (which is not natural at all, as there is no such thing as a canola plant), eating margarine (which is made from trans fats) and pushing down hot dogs. Eating like this will certainly create severe nutrient deficiencies and cause illness.

However, a proper approach to the ketogenic diet, which includes lots of fatty cuts from high-quality meat produced from animals that are raised organically, nuts, leafy green vegetables, dairy, butter, olive oil and avocados, the diet is actually very nutrient dense. In fact, you will be consuming much more vitamins and minerals than in a typical American diet.

Lower cholesterol and risk of heart disease

The scary fact behind heart disease is that it is caused by eating carbs, not fats. Increasing research is revealing that heart disease rates are higher in people who eat a lot of carbs, even though traditional advice is that people with risk factors for heart disease should limit their fat intake. Carbs raise blood triglycerides, the dangerous fats that float through your bloodstream and can cause blockages when they build up to dangerous levels. Additionally, growing evidence suggests that carbs, not fats, raise the bad LDL cholesterol that can also clog arteries. The more carbs you eat, the higher your risk of heart disease.

There is a lot of misunderstanding about how cholesterol actually works. It is necessary for bodily function and is produced naturally; the body's cholesterol levels are actually affected very little by the foods that we eat. The carriers of the cholesterol are either the high-density lipoproteins (HDL) or low-density lipoproteins (LDL), which are determined by the foods that we eat. Eating a lot of cholesterol doesn't increase chances of heart disease.

Triglycerides are the fats that are stored in your fat cells but can also accumulate in the bloodstream. They can also accumulate in the liver, leading to fatty liver disease. They are produced from glucose, so the best way to lower your triglycerides is to severely restrict the carbs that you are consuming. Numerous studies show that a high-fat diet, as compared with a high-carb diet, is very effective at lowering levels of triglycerides, as long as the fats consumed are healthy.

Healthy fats actually purge the bad triglycerides and LDL from your bloodstream, thereby lowering the risk factors for heart disease. They clean up the blood

Increased energy

Insulin, which is secreted whenever carbs are consumed so that cells are able to absorb the energy, causes fatigue and drowsiness. This is why you often feel sleepy after eating a large meal. Additionally, glucose is not very efficient at creating energy and leaves a lot of waste products, thereby exacerbating fatigue. People on carb-rich diets tend to sleep much more than people on high-fat diets because they just don't have energy.

Once insulin levels are lowered and the body is adjusted to burning ketones instead of glucose, energy levels increase dramatically. Some people on the ketogenic diet report needing less sleep and are able to thrive on just six hours, whereas doctors recommend seven to eight. Interestingly, traditional cultures that consume high-fat diets also sleep closer to six hours, suggesting that there may be a link between eating a high-fat diet and needing less sleep.

Balanced hormones

At the heart of many diseases are imbalanced hormones. Insulin is one of the most proliferate hormones in the human body and problems with its levels immediately affect other hormones, including sex hormones, satiety hormones and hunger hormones. Stabilizing and permanently lowering insulin levels leads to balanced hormones all across the body. This is why people with metabolic syndrome, PCOS, acne and other hormonal problems benefit immensely from the ketogenic diet.

Decreased inflammation

Inflammation is the body's natural response to infection and foreign invaders. When you cut your finger, the skin around the cut quickly becomes red and inflamed, as your body is responding to the microbes that may be entering. While some inflammation is good as an acute response, many people live in a state of chronic inflammation caused by poor diet. Inflamed tissues can develop scar tissue and be unable to function properly. Inflamed joints become painful and inflamed blood vessels cause heart disease.

A ketogenic diet has been shown to substantially decrease inflammation over the long term. The body is still able to use inflammation as an acute response to foreign invaders, but it is no longer a chronic issue.

Chapter Four:
Basics of Planning Meals

To know what you have to eat on a ketogenic diet, you will have to understand caloric requirements and content and fats, protein and carbohydrates. You have to understand their different kinds and the different roles they perform for your body. Furthermore, you need to know what macronutrients are good and harmful for your health so that you can build a diet that is both ketogenic and healthy.

In addition, for the ketogenic diet to work, you need to remove all packaged and processed foods from your diet. It should consist of high-quality, healthy fats, fiber-rich carbohydrates with the least net carbohydrates (total carbohydrates minus fiber) as possible.

Important: Before you create a plan for your ketogenic diet, you need to consult first a nutritionist or a medical professional to determine the number of daily calories you require based on your age, height, weight, gender and age as well as body fat percentage. This would make sure that you are not merely guessing in setting the calories you need for your body.
Fats

In the 1980s, doctors, nutritionists and public health officials campaigned to the public that fats are not a part of a healthy diet. They said that fat is the cause of weight gain and heart disease. However, this is only true for the bad quality of fat in food. Fats play a critical role in providing a denser caloric content per gram compared to proteins and carbohydrates. Because of this, fat can provide adequate energy when food is scarce or when a person is unable to consume large amounts of food.

Fats

Fats in your diet contain mixtures of fatty acids. These nutrients contain a mixture of saturated and unsaturated fats. Saturated fats are most abundant in animal-derived fats while unsaturated fats are most abundant in plant-derived ones. Other than the dense caloric property fats, it provides fatty acids that regulate inflammation in the body. It carries fat-soluble vitamins. Lastly, it provides texture and flavor to your meal, making it more satisfying to your appetite.

Fats to avoid
Excess Saturated Fat

The key to having healthy fat consumption is to minimize the consumption of food rich in saturated fats. Although your body needs both kinds of fat, saturated fats from foods derived from plants are enough to provide you with your saturated fat needs. Having high levels of saturated fat in your body leads to heart and cardiovascular disease.

Moreover, it is not enough to replace saturated fat-rich foods with fat-free food products as these are high in carbohydrates and increase the risk of the same disease mentioned. Here's a list of foods rich in saturated fat that you should avoid:

- Fat from processed meats like sausages, ham and burgers

- Fatty meat
- Hard cheeses
- Butter
- Lard
- Ghee
- Palm Oil

Trans Fat

Trans fat, or trans-unsaturated fats, occur in nature albeit in small amounts, but they are also widely manufactured commercially from vegetable fats for use in various manufactured food products. This is created by adding hydrogen gas to vegetable oil, which causes the oil to become solid at room temperature.

The reason why food manufacturers create and use this is to make food have a longer shelf life or have a better flavor. These fats contribute to insulin resistance and unbalance your cholesterol levels by increasing the bad and decreasing the good.

Manufactured trans-fat can be found in food products like:

- Baked goods like cake, pie crusts and crackers and ready-made frosting
- Snacks like packaged microwave popcorn and potato, corn and tortilla chips.
- Fried food due to the oil used in the cooking process
- Refrigerator dough like canned biscuits, cinnamon rolls and frozen pizza crusts
- Non-dairy coffee creamer
- Margarine
- In food labels, trans fat can also be listed as shortening, hydrogenated oil, partially hydrogenated oil and hydrogenated vegetable oil.

Fats you can eat

The key to having a healthy ketogenic diet is choosing wisely the fats you include in your diet without exceeding your calorie requirement. The important part of this diet is to consume the correct ratio of macronutrients. You need between five and ten percent of your calories to be from net carbs, 15 and 30 percent from protein and 65 to 75 percent or more from fat to be able to benefit from the ketones that get produced by the liver.

Is there a right amount of fat intake with a ketogenic diet? This amount will vary for everybody. It depends on your goals. You don't need to count your calories or fat intake on a keto diet since eating foods that are naturally low in carbs keep your feeling full longer.

Studies have shown that fats and proteins are the most filling nutrients and carbs are the least. Fats contribute to a steady energy supply and don't cause insulin spikes. This is the reason you don't have cravings, mood swings or fluctuating energy. For some, counting calories and tracking macros can help break through a stubborn weight loss plateau.

The macronutrient ratio isn't all you need to consider. You need to understand what fats are good for you and what can be detrimental to your health. The different qualities and types of fat make a difference. When figuring out what fats and oil to use, here are some simple rules to follow:

When cooking, use saturated fats. These fats have gotten a bad rap as being bad for us. We have heard that cholesterol and saturated fats cause obesity and heart disease for the past 50 years. This lipid hypothesis was created by Ancel Keys' fraudulent and flawed research. Saturated fats can be found in palm oil, coconut oil, eggs, tallow, lard, ghee, butter, cream and red meat. These oils have a high smoke point, long shelf life and are the most stable. Use these for cooking. The majority of fats need to come from monounsaturated and saturated fats.

Try adding medium chain triglycerides to your diet. These are fats that can be easily digested. These triglycerides can be found in coconut oil. They act differently when ingested and are sent straight to the liver. They can be immediately used for energy. They are found in palm oil and butter in lesser quantities. Medium chain triglycerides are used by bodybuilders and athletes to improve their performance and help them lose fat. If your body is able to handle pure MCT oil without causing any stomach problems, you should be able to find it as a supplement.

Include monounsaturated fatty acids. Omega 9, oleic acid or monounsaturated fatty acids can be found in nuts, beef, olives and avocados. These help to prevent heart disease. Consuming monounsaturated fatty acids can give better serum lipid profiles. Monounsaturated fatty acids like macadamia nut, avocado and extra virgin olive oil are the best for using cold like drizzling over a finished a meal.

You can use unsaturated fats. You do not heat them. Our body needs omega 6s, Omega 3s and polyunsaturated fatty acids. These are common in our everyday lives and we consume too many. These fatty acids are called poly because they have many double bonds. When these bonds are heated, they react with oxygen to form compounds that are harmful like free radicals. This process increases inflammation and makes free radicals that put us at risk for cancer and heart disease. Polyunsaturated fats are not stable and should not be used for high heat cooking. Avocado oil, flaxseed oil, sesame oil, nut oils and extra virgin olive oil are best to use cold. Flaxseed oil shouldn't be heated and needs to be refrigerated. Olive, Macadamia and avocado oil can be used for light cooking or for finishing the meal.

The Omega 6 fatty acids and omega 3 fatty acids need to be balanced. Both of these are polyunsaturated fatty acids and are essential. Studies have shown that most diets are deficient in omega 3s. The omega 6 and omega 3 ratio is unfavorable between 15 to 1 and 17 to 1. This ratio needs to be balanced at one to one. It will be better for your health if you can get this ratio as close to one to one as possible. Studies have shown that eating more omega 6 and lower omega 3s are known to cause inflammatory diseases, autoimmune disorders, stroke and cardiovascular disease. Reducing your intake of omega 6s might protect you against these diseases. You are probably getting enough omega 6s so try to focus on increasing the intake of omega 3s by eating macadamia nuts, walnuts, grass-fed meat, fermented cod liver oil and wild salmon.

Your Omega 3 intake should come from animals. Omega 3 is either long chain that is found in seafood and fish or short chain that is found in nuts and seeds. While Eicosapentaenoic acid or EPA and docosahexaenoic acid or DHA affect omega 6s to 3s ratios, the alpha-linoleic acid or ALA needs to be converted to DHA or EPA. Our bodies can't convert ALA to DHA or EPA. This is why you need to get the omega 3s from the meat of animals. When buying meat, find grass fed to get the most omega 3s. Meat from animals that have been grain fed had very low omega 3s but packed full of omega 6s.

Be aware of shelf life, oxidation rate and smoke point. A higher smoke point is better. Oils that have a high smoke point can be used to cook foods at high temperatures. If you heat the oil above its smoke point, this can damage the oil and release free radicals.

Having an oxidation rate that is slow is better. The oxidation rate increases when it gets heated to its smoking point. These can also oxidize on the shelf. Metals like copper and iron can also cause them to oxidize. Any oil is capable of going rancid while sitting on in the pantry. This will load them with free radicals. Higher saturated fat oils will last longer around 12 to 24 months. Oils that are high in monounsaturated fats will last about six to twelve months. Polyunsaturated fats have a shelf life of about two to six months.

Stay away from all unhealthy oils. Corn, grapeseed, soybean, canola, cottonseed, safflower, sunflower oils, trans fats, partially hydrogenated oils, hydrogenated oils, margarine and processed vegetable oils are all bad for your health. Processed oils and trans fatty acids:

- Are oxidized with high heat and created free radicals.
- These are created from genetically modified seeds.
- Are pro-inflammatory and bad for your gut.
- Eating trans fats raises the risk of developing coronary heart disease.

- Consuming trans fats will affect cholesterol levels negatively. They reduce the level of HDL or good cholesterol and increase the level of LDL or bad cholesterol.
- Can cause an increased risk of cancer.

All of these fats exist within nature and occur during the processing of polyunsaturated fatty acids in food production. These naturally occurring trans fats are beneficial when you compare them to artificial trans fats. These natural trans fats can be found in the meat of animals that have been grass fed and dairy products.

Metabolic poison refers to artificial trans fats. Get these out of your diet by staying away from any food that contains partially hydrogenated or hydrogenated oils. You can find these in French fries, crackers, cookies and margarine.

Proteins

Most foods contain some amount of protein including vegetables and grain. Foods that have substantial amounts of protein are meat from animals, dairy products, beans and nuts. It can provide energy for your body. However, it is not its primary purpose.

When broken down into amino acids, the body would use this to create its own proteins intended for various purposes. With the 20 amino acids that your body would need, it can create an infinite number of proteins like enzymes for chemical reactions, hormones for triggering organs, collagen for bone structure and antibodies for the immune system. Your body's proteins are constantly broken down and re-synthesized to build more proteins. Most of the amino acids from broken down protein are reused, but some are lost and must be replaced through your diet.

Proteins to avoid

What you have to watch out for in proteins in your diet is eating too much of it. The excess protein that you got from your food would be converted to sugar and then fat which would be stored for later use. It could also increase the stimulation of your mTOR, which increases your chances of developing cancer. Additionally, the excess protein requires your body to remove more nitrogen, a by-product of protein digestion, which stresses out your kidneys.

Proteins to eat

Moderate consumption of high-quality protein is the key. Protein for a ketogenic diet should come from a variety of plant and animal sources. Meat products should be lean to avoid adding fats that are mostly saturated. The suggested protein for a ketogenic diet varies from person to person. Generally, the recommended daily protein of 0.8g per pound of lean body mass for a sedentary lifestyle, 0.8 to 1g per pound of body mass for a lightly active lifestyle and 1.0 – 1.2g for a highly active lifestyle.

Carbohydrates

Carbohydrates are the starches, sugars and fibers found in the food that we eat. The sugars and starches we eat are broken down into its simplest chemical forms while, as it is indigestible, fibers just pass through the digestive system.

Sugars, also known as simple carbohydrates, are found in fruit and vegetables that can be broken down to sucrose and/ or fructose. Starches, also known as complex carbohydrates, are found in grains that can be broken down into glucose (also known as blood sugar).

Of all these carbohydrates, glucose is the most preferred as it can be readily circulated from the digestive process into various parts of the body. Meanwhile, fructose can only be used for energy by the liver and sucrose is further broken down into glucose and fructose.

The role of fiber: The most common question with low carb dieters is: Do I need to include fiber when counting my carbs?

Let's see: Some soluble gets absorbed, but humans, in general, don't possess all the needed enzymes to digest fibers and then be able to get calories out of it. Because of this, fiber doesn't affect blood sugar or ketosis. You can try to get between 20 and 25 grams of net carbs or less than 50 grams of total carbs.

If the fiber isn't counted, the carbs are referred to as net carbs. Calculating net carbs can reduce how high fiber foods are impacted and allow you to eat them. This is a common argument for those who criticize the low carb diet because it lacks fiber. An important note is that fiber does not negate carbs. They are just not counted. You can't just mix some flax meal into pasta.

In Canada and the United States, food labels include fiber with the carbohydrate values in a term known as total carbs. This calculates carbs by using an indirect method. Carbs get calculated after the ash, water, fat and protein has been measured out. To figure net carbs, you subtract the amount of fiber from the total carbs. This type of food label isn't used all over the world. In Oceania, Australia and Europe, their food labels don't include fiber. They calculate carbs using a direct method. The carbs listed on their food labels will just be net carbs. Don't worry about where you buy the food but think about the country it came from.

Is there a way to be certain about the amounts of net carbs? You can follow these rules:

- Total carbs will never be less than the amount of fiber.
- The total carbs minus the fiber is never going to be less than the sugar. For example, lactose + other sugar + sugars = net carbs.
- Calories that come from carbs (without fiber) + calories that come from protein + calories that come from fat

= total kcal

Although fiber cannot be digested, it plays a key role in the digestion of carbohydrates in the body. It slows down the rate of digestion and absorption of carbohydrates, thereby preventing the blood sugar from rapidly shooting up. Aside from that, fibers provide food for your beneficial gut bacteria, improving digestion and bowel movement.

Fibers also contain phytochemicals like lycopene, lutein and indole-3-carbinol. These stimulate the immune system, fight free radicals and protect and repair the DNA.

Carbs to avoid

Refined Carbohydrates

Refined carbohydrates are whole plants or plant-derived products that have been processed to remove everything except the highly digestible carbohydrate in it. To refine carbohydrates, the whole sugar, plant, or grain is stripped of its fibers, vitamins and minerals. This is done usually as other parts of the plant cannot be digested by the body or to make the plant easier to manipulate into mixtures and food products.

Refining removes everything including valuable natural vitamins and minerals and, to circumvent the lack of micronutrients, manufacturers add synthetic vitamins and minerals back into the carbohydrates.

Refined carbohydrates in an average person's diet usually come from:

- White flour from white bread, pasta and other food products containing it.
- White rice that is usually "enriched" with the synthetic vitamins and minerals.
- Sugar from bread, pastries, sweets and breakfast cereals.
- Sugar and High Fructose Corn Syrup from sodas and other sweetened beverages.
- Sugar from any other food product that has been added before consumption like ketchup and mustard.

With the fibers removed from these carbohydrates, your body digests it quickly. This results in a rapid absorption of broken down carbohydrates into your body. Particularly, in the case of glucose, your blood sugar rises so fast that your body would have to release insulin to signal your body to start storing it. This causes a volatile and erratic volume of blood sugar in your system. This usually manifests to sluggishness and/ or hunger even though you just had a heavy carbohydrate meal. If your body experiences this often, it will pave the way for insulin resistance and, eventually, Type 2 Diabetes.

On the other hand, fructose from refined carbohydrates that are used as sweeteners and other forms of added sugars have compound said harmful effects. Excess consumption of foods containing added fructose could lead to:

- Visceral fat gain
- Increased uric acid levels leading to gout and high blood pressure,
- Insulin resistance
- Leptin resistance that disturbs body fat regulation and contributing to obesity.

High Fructose Corn Syrup

High Fructose Corn Syrup (HFCS) is a refined carbohydrate that comes from corn. It is a sugar substitute that is a hundred times sweeter than sucrose, the common sugar. Since it costs substantially less and is not affected by fluctuating import prices, it is a very good alternative for sugar. It started gaining popularity during the 1970s when it began being used by food manufacturers. Its use in different food products steadily rose since then.

The incidences of obesity are higher in countries where its use is prevalent. Add to that the fact, that in the 1980s up to the present date, obesity rates in the United States steadily rose, matching the trend of rising availability of HFCS in food products.

Moreover, studies have shown that, even in moderate consumption, HFCS is a major cause of various diseases like heart disease, obesity, cancer, dementia and liver failure. Even though HFCS is used as a substitute for sucrose, the body does not respond to it in the same way.

Carbs to Eat

In a ketogenic diet, you must stick to protein, vegetables, fats and oils, full-fat dairy and nuts and seeds of your diet. From these items, you will already be able to get the fiber that you need for your diet. Adding any kind of grain or sugar in your diet would only prevent you from reaching your goals in the diet. However, if you want to have your fix of carbohydrates, you can use flour substitutes like coconut flour and flaxseed meal.

For carbohydrates in a Standard Ketogenic Diet, the maximum daily intake is 5% of total daily calorie intake. Refer to the net carbs of the food items given in preparing the carbohydrates for your meals.

Beverages

The ketogenic diet is very particular in controlling what goes into your body. Drinking alcohol, sweetened beverages and fruit juices would mess up your sugar levels and could push you further from reaching ketosis. Therefore, you must only drink water and coffee and tea with no sweeteners, creamer and dairy. Anything else other than these three should not be drunk.

The ketogenic diet causes a natural diuretic effect. Dehydration is common for many people who are just starting on this diet. If you get bladder pain or urinary tract infections, you need to be prepared. The normal eight glasses that are recommended for you to drink - you need to drink those and then more. Our body consists of two-thirds water. Drink at least a gallon of water everyday, as hydration is extremely important.

Many choose keto friendly coffee or tea of the mornings to give their energy a boost with added fats. It is good; just remember to avoid flavored beverages as much as possible. This becomes amplified with caffeine as too much may hamper your weight loss. Try to only have about two caffeinated beverages each day.

Some examples of beverages you can have with your keto diet are:

- Water: This is your go-to for hydration. You may have sparkling or plain water.
- Broth: This is loaded with nutrients and vitamins. Most important, it gives your energy a boost by replenishing your electrolytes.
- Coffee: This will improve your mental focus and has weight loss benefits.
- Tea: This has the same effects as coffee. Some people don't like tea. Try either green or black tea.
- Almond or coconut milk: Use the unsweetened versions in a carton from your grocery store to replace your favorite dairy drink.
- Diet soda: You need to reduce or completely stop drinking these. These can cause sugar cravings and insulin spikes.
- Flavoring: These little packets are flavored with stevia or sucralose and are fine. You can also add orange, lime and lemon to your water.
- Alcohol: If you need your alcohol, choose hard liquor. Wine and beer will be too high in carbs to drink. Frequent consumption of alcohol will slow down your weight loss.

Most people like to keep themselves accountable for the actions by creating a challenge for themselves. Try using a 32-ounce water bottle and place four hair-ties around it. Every time you finish a bottle, take away one hair tie. Keep on drinking until there aren't any left.

Recommended Foods

Below is a comprehensive list of the common food items that are recommended for your ketogenic diet. Each item has information of its nutritional value arranged as such: "amount of item/ calories/fat / net carbohydrates/protein."

Protein

The best proteins for a ketogenic diet are those that are pasture-raised and grass-fed. This will minimize your exposure from bacteria and growth hormones. Choose darker poultry meat and fatty fish that are rich in omega 3. Balance out your protein portions in your meals with fats and oil to aid in its digestion.

- Ground beef (4oz, 80/ 20 / 280 / 23g / 0g / 20g)
- Ribeye steak (4oz / 330 / 25g / 0g / 27g)
- Bacon (4oz / 519 / 51g / 0g / 13g)
- Pork chop (4oz / 286 / 18g / 0g / 30g)
- Chicken thigh (4oz / 250 / 20g / 0g / 17g)
- Chicken breast (4oz / 125 / 1g / 0 / 26g)
- Salmon (4oz / 236 / 15g / 0g / 23g)
- Ground lamb (4oz / 319 / 27g / 0g / 19g)
- Liver (4oz / 135 / 5g / 0g / 19g)
- Egg (1 large / 70 / 5g / 0.5g / 6g)
- Almond butter (2tbsp / 180 / 16g / 4g/ 6)

Vegetables and Fruit

Cruciferous vegetables that are grown above ground, leafy and green are the best for a ketogenic diet. On the other hand, vegetables that grow below ground should be eaten in moderation as these have higher carbohydrate amounts.

- Cabbage (6 oz. / 43g / 0g / 6g / 2g)
- Cauliflower (6 oz. / 40 / 0g / 6g / 5g)
- Broccoli (6 oz. / 58 / 1g / 7g / 5g)
- Spinach (6 oz. / 24 / 0g / 1g / 3g)
- Romaine Lettuce (6 oz. / 29 / 1g / 2g / 2g)
- Green Bell Pepper (6 oz. / 33 / 0g / 5g / 1g)
- Baby Bella Mushrooms (6 oz. / 40 / 0g / 4g / 6g)
- Green Beans (6 oz. / 26 / 0g / 4g / 2g)
- Yellow Onion (6 oz. / 68 / 0g / 12g / 2g)
- Blackberries (6 oz. / 73 / 1g / 8g / 2g)
- Raspberries (6 oz. / 88 / 1g / 8g / 2g)

Dairy Products

If available, give preference to raw and organic dairy products. Avoid highly processed dairy as these have a higher amount of carbohydrates than raw/ organic ones. Also avoid products with higher carbohydrate levels.

- Heavy cream (1 oz. / 100g / 12g / 0g / 0g)
- Greek yogurt (1 oz. / 28g / 1g / 1g / 3g)
- Mayonnaise (1 oz. / 180g / 20g / 0g / 0g)
- Half n' half (1 oz. / 40 / 4g / 1g / 1g)
- Cottage cheese (1 oz. / 25g / 1g / 1g / 4g)
- Cream Cheese (1 oz. / 94 / 9g / 1g / 2g)
- Mascarpone (1 oz. / 120g / 13g / 0g / 2g)
- Mozzarella (1 oz. / 70 / 5g / 1g / 5g)
- Brie (1 oz. / 95 / 8g / 0g / 6g)
- Aged Cheddar (1 oz. / 110 / 9g / 0g / 7g)

- Parmesan (1 oz. / 110 / 7g / 1g / 10g)

Nuts and Seeds

These are best when roasted to remove any anti-nutrients present. These can be added to add flavor or texture to your meals.

- Macadamia Nuts (2 oz. / 407 / 43g / 3g / 4g)
- Brazil Nuts (2 oz. / 373 / 37g / 3g / 8g)
- Pecans (2 oz. / 392 / 41g / 3g / 5g)
- Almonds (2 oz. / 328 / 28g / 5g / 12g)
- Hazelnuts (2 oz. / 356 / 36g / 3g / 9g)

Nut and Seed Flours

These can be used as a substitute for regular flour in making baked and dessert recipes.

- Almond Flour (2 oz. / 324 / 28g / 6g / 12g)
- Coconut Flour (2 oz. / 120 / 4g / 6g / 4g)
- Chia Seed Meal (2 oz. / 265 / 17g / 3g / 8g)
- Flaxseed Meal (2 oz. / 224 / 18g / 1g / 8g)
- Unsweetened Coconut (2 oz. / 445 / 40g / 8g / 4g)

Getting Started

Before you even get started on this diet, you must first decide on your goal and why you're doing this. Are you looking to lose unhealthy body fat? Are you looking to therapeutically heal a degenerative disease? Are you aiming to change your lifestyle? Whatever the case may be, you must first decide why you're going to do this diet. Without clarity on your goal, you can't choose an approach for your diet and can't properly plan for how to do it.

Get Yourself Tested

You must first determine that your body can undergo the diet and the massive adjustments it would make. You also have to determine your body fat percentage, weight and other relevant data to create your personal macronutrient mix via keto calculators available online.

Get Support

You have to talk to your family, especially if they live in the same house as you. If you're the only one who's doing this diet, your family might misunderstand when you can't eat like them, or you have a different food from theirs. Moreover, on the first few weeks, you might miss out on the next birthday party or family gathering just to distance yourself from tempting carbohydrates.

Other than that, your family can also help you in keeping you in line with the diet. They can call you out whenever you're about to slip from it. Also, if you have children, you can make it fun for them by making them your carbohydrate police at home. If you live alone, you can get support by joining community forums online.

Plan the meals that you will have

Even before you shop for your ketogenic groceries, you must first know the meals you will be eating beforehand. This would save you time and would make sure that you have the right ingredients ready for making ketogenic meals. This would reduce the excuses you can think of to just nibble on carbohydrates or say, "it would just be one meal."

Also, this gives you the opportunity to research for recipes that you might like. Other than that, after you find recipes that you like, you can plan out your meals for your next run to the grocery. Clean out the Carbohydrates out of Your House

This is the best way of preventing yourself from slipping up and "accidentally" eating that cookie. If there are no food items in your house to tempt you, you cannot be tempted to eat what you shouldn't. This would surely help you, as the first few months are the hardest due to your body still adapting to ketosis.

Undergo an Adaptation Period

To make the ketogenic diet easier for you, you could slowly ease into it by either fasting intermittently to or cut your carbohydrates. By fasting intermittently, you have 16 hours wherein you don't eat anything and only 8 hours wherein you can. This forces your body to enter a state of fasting and you get used to having your blood sugar into a fasted state.

On the other hand, by cutting your calories, your body is being trained to get used to having smaller portions of carbohydrates that it used to. Like in intermittent fasting, it decreases the shock of having very little carbohydrates in your diet. One practice is by limiting daily net carbohydrates to only 30 grams for 6 days in a week and having a high carbohydrate meal for dinner of the 7th day. This is repeated for every 7 days for at least 4 weeks.

Chapter Five:
Setting up a Plan

In this section, I will familiarize you with some practical aspects that you might need to know about to set up a plan.

Keto Shopping List

There are plenty of keto foods out there. Here is a list to help you get started with your first shopping trip:

Vegetables:

- Asparagus
- Broccoli
- Cabbage
- Pickles
- Black Olives
- Green Olives
- Sauerkraut
- Cauliflower
- Spinach, fresh and canned
- Green onions
- Iceberg Lettuce
- Mushrooms
- Okra
- Spaghetti Squash
- Yellow Onions

- Zucchini
- Yellow Squash
- Leeks
- Canned Green Beans

Fruit:

- Any berry
- Rhubarb
- Tomatoes in moderation
- Lemons
- Limes
- Avocado
- Coconut
- Figs
- Watermelon
- Cherries
- Pomegranate
- Papaya
- Raisins
- Plums
- Clementine
- Apple
- Guava

Dairy:

- Full Fat Milk
- Full Fat Greek Yogurt
- Mayonnaise
- Heavy Whipping Cream
- Sour Cream

Cheeses:

- Swiss
- String Cheese
- Parmesan
- Mozzarella
- Monterey Jack
- Goat Cheese
- Feta
- Cream Cheese
- Cottage Cheese
- Colby
- Cheddar
- Brie
- Blue

Meats:

- Beef
- Chicken
- Pork
- Turkey
- Tuna
- Salmon
- Cod
- Flounder
- Tilapia
- Shrimp
- Scallops
- Lobster

Spices:

- All herbs and spices

Dressings and Sauces:

- Lime Juice
- Lemon Juice
- Italian
- Ranch
- Blue Cheese
- Brown and Yellow Mustard
- Worcestershire Sauce
- Vinegar
- Soy Sauce
- Sugar-Free Syrup
- Sugar-Free Ketchup
- Low-Carb Salsa

Liquids:

- Protein Shakes
- Unsweetened Tea
- Coffee (can add heavy cream)
- Almond Milk
- Cashew Milk
- Coconut Milk

Oils and Fats:

- Sunflower Oil
- Sesame Oil
- Peanut Oil

- Olive Oil
- Mayonnaise
- Coconut Oil
- Bacon Fat
- Butter

Baking and Cooking:

- Cocoa Power
- Chia Seeds
- Flax Seeds
- Flax Meal
- Almond Meal/Flour
- Coconut Flakes
- Coconut Flour

Sweeteners:

- Xylitol
- Stevia Drops
- Erythritol

Evaluate Your Keto Diet Experience

With your meal plan and recipes ready to go and your mind ready for the diet, you begin. In the first week, things immediately start to get uncomfortable and your energy seems to have dropped to almost nonexistent levels. This shouldn't come as a surprise since this is normal for anyone and it is simply signs of your body being in a transition.

Common Side Effects

With any change to your diet, it is normal to have some side effects as your body begins to adapt to the new way you are eating. When doing a ketogenic diet, the body must switch the fuel source from glucose to fat stores. This can cause some of the following side effects:

Keto Flu

With your body used to only breaking down carbohydrates and using it for energy, it had built up numerous enzymes dedicated to this process. Because of the body's dependence on carbohydrates, it neglected the production of enzymes for dealing with fats. Then, your body is suddenly dealing with a lack of glucose and constant supply of fats, which triggers the body to start producing enzymes for using fat as fuel.

However, this would take time and not only one or two days. The first few weeks on a keto diet is challenging for some and easy for others. Your body is used to relying on glucose for energy, so it needs to switch to using ketones for fuel. This can result in brain fog but disappears when the body gets adapted. This adaptation takes about four weeks, but the side effects disappear sooner. Around the end of the first week, it is normal to feel some flu-like symptoms like cravings, insomnia, racing heart when lying down, fatigue, dizziness and brain fog. You can lessen these effects by gradually lowering your carb intake over a few weeks. If you decide to just right into a keto diet, just remember to get plenty of fluids and salts. This will keep you from feeling lousy.

This is called Keto Flu and is a natural transitional response of your body. This usually happens during the first week of your ketogenic diet. In this state, you will experience headaches, mental fogginess, dizziness and aggravation. These ailments are due to your electrolytes being eliminated in your body because ketones have a diuretic effect. To counteract this, you should drink plenty of water and increase the sodium in your body.

Curing the Keto Flu

The keto flu will vary with each person. Many find the symptoms are worst in the first week. Some find they linger for weeks on end. There are some tricks you can do to shorten your flu time:

- Eat more fats: This is a common method used to combat the keto flu. Your body needs energy. It isn't getting it from sugar and carbs, so it needs to get it from what you are eating. Eat lots of healthy fats like lard, tallow, ghee, olive oil and coconut oil. To stay in ketosis, you need to consume plenty of fats. Adding MCT oil can boost your ketone level. This will help your brain feel better.
- Eat more calories: It is easy to not eat enough when you begin a low carb diet. Many just cut out the carbs without increasing other food intakes. They get confused about what they can eat since they are used to eating bread, rice and pasta.
- Exercise: This might be the last thing you are thinking about right now. Studies show that exercise helps you to become more metabolically flexible. This means that your body can switch between carbs and ketones for energy easily. People that don't experience the keto flu for long are more metabolically flexible because they can switch between ketones and carbs.

Bad Breath

This is sometimes called keto breath. It can happen as you go into ketosis. Ketones get released into the breath, sweat and urine. Acetone is one form of a ketone that is released in the breath and can cause a metallic taste in the mouth. This is temporary and will disappear after a couple of weeks. If this becomes a problem, sugar-free breath fresheners or gum can help. You can increase your oral hygiene by using mouthwash and brushing your teeth more often.

Leg Cramps

Developing muscle cramps might be possible with the keto diet. These can sometimes be rather bothersome. The cause of cramps is a condition called hyponatremia. This happens when salt levels are too low. Stay hydrated and add salt to the diet.

Loss of Salts

There will be changes in your fluid balance in the first few weeks on the keto diet. This happens as the body uses up the stored sugars that in turn release water into the blood that gets flushed out through the urine. When fluids get passed out, salts in the body will become depleted. Keep yourself hydrated. Water is best, but coffee and tea are fine as long as they aren't extremely milky. Make sure you have plenty of salt, so you won't experience side effects like wooziness and headaches. You can add sea salt to your food and drink bone or vegetable bouillons and broths. Magnesium and potassium are important salts, too.

If you are eating natural, healthy foods like vegetables, dairy, fish, meat and nuts, you shouldn't have any problems getting the potassium and magnesium you need.

Bowel Habit Change

A keto diet can cause constipation. The body's gut bacteria need to adapt to be able to handle the different foods and the different amounts of food. Bowel habits usually improve in a couple of weeks. If they don't, make sure you are getting enough fiber. Drink lots of water and increase the amounts of seeds, nuts, legumes and fibrous vegetables.

Loss of Energy

The biggest misconception of the keto diet is the lack of glucose will deplete the body of its energy. Keeping steady energy is more challenging with a standard diet because it fluctuates with blood sugar.

Eating lower carbs doesn't prevent the sugar level rollercoaster. Once the body gets into ketosis, the body begins to draw energy from its fat stores. The liver begins to create the amount of glucose the body needs.

By cutting down on carbs, the body will find it easier to regulate energy and sugar level. You might notice a dip in energy while adapting to the diet; this should pass in a few weeks.

Poor Physical Performance

Due to low levels of blood sugar, your physical performance will drop. This is only for the short term and your body will eventually adapt to it. However, if you have to always be on top of your performance, it will be beneficial for you if you adopt either the Cyclic or Targeted Ketogenic Diet. These two approaches will provide you the energy for your physical activities and, at the same time, enable you to have a ketogenic diet.

Other than that, you may also experience cramps, constipation and heart palpitations. These are easily remedied by your proper hydration and by eating foods with good sources of micronutrients. There is nothing to be alarmed when you experience these effects. In fact, they tell you that your body is adjusting to a state of ketosis.

These side effects are normally temporary and can be remedied.

Signs that you've reached Ketosis
- Bad breath due to acetone, a ketone being expelled through your mouth or urine.
- Dry mouth and increased thirst due to ketones being diuretics.
- Increased urination

What to watch out for

It is important to keep track of your ketones to make sure that your body is responding to the diet and to prevent ketoacidosis. It is when the ketones in your body approach dangerous levels. Although it is easy to assume that ketones can reach high levels, this is simply not true and is, in fact, a rare occurrence.

It is still important to regularly keep track of your ketones. This can easily be done and no need for laboratory tests to be done. Ketone testing can easily be done through urine strips, breath ketone analyzers and blood ketone meter.

Keeping up Motivation

Beginning a new diet is exciting. You see all the transformation pictures online and you start to see how your body will change, also. Sticking to a keto diet until it becomes your lifestyle gets challenging. If you can stick to the keto diet for a few months, you will get the results of more energy, mental clarity and loss of body fat. Here are some techniques to help you:

1. Start small. It is tempting to go all in in the beginning. Your motivation will be high and we have a tendency to push ourselves to the limit. We think we have to cook all our meals at home instead of going out to eat. We

have to join a gym and work out for hours five days a week. This will cause the body to crash and burn and the result is stopping the diet completely. The answer to this is the pick a small change that is easy to commit to. If you want to change your whole diet, start by changing your breakfast. Don't go to the gym for hours every day just do 15 minutes two times a week. By starting small, it will be impossible not to do it. Create the habit first and then increase it once you have gained traction.

2. Eat the same things. The reason many people don't stick to a diet is that they are looking for a variety each day. If they get stressed out or their willpower is tested, they just go to a fast food restaurant. If they can learn to eat the same meals each day, it will reduce the likelihood of cheating since you already know what you are going to eat. Repeat the same three or four meal over and over. Try variety on the weekends.

3. Take some food with you. We might not always be around keto friendly food. It might be a family gathering or a party at work. The temptation is everywhere. The key here is controlling your environment. Pack a lunchbox or backpack full of keto-friendly snacks to take with you wherever you go. If you begin to feel tempted grab a handful and eat away. This might save you from cheating on your diet.

4. Make success rewarding. Most people know how to lose weight. Having a true reason to change is the answer, not more information. Use positive reinforcements to help. Set realistic weight loss goals for yourself like losing ten pounds in 30 days. Think of something that you have wanted to do for a long time like taking a trip someplace you've never been or spending the day at a spa. You can only do this if you reach your weight loss goal.

5. Never try to be perfect. Stay focused on the progress, not perfection. Be okay with grabbing a non-keto snack every now and then. Too many have

quit reaching for their goal because they think they have failed. We are all human. To err is human. The real failure here is just giving up.

Long-Term Tips

No matter how much you love the ketogenic diet, there are family reunions, parties and other events that can easily derail your best-laid plans. Holidays and birthdays can be particularly difficult, as you are surrounded by sweet and savory dishes that bring back fond memories. Being surrounded by relatives and friends who lovingly prepared all of the food can make resisting even more difficult. Having to prepare food separately from what you feed your family can be difficult. Additionally, you are probably finding that the ketogenic diet takes a lot of commitment. Food preparation, storage and grocery shopping can take vastly larger amounts of time than before. Plus, it costs more than eating a high-carb diet. Here are some tips to help you stay on the ketogenic diet long-term.

Plan ahead

Planning your meals in advance is a strategic way to manage a busy schedule while sticking to a healthy eating plan. Prepare your grocery list before you go to the store so that you don't forget anything that you need. Having to make an extra grocery trip during the week can easily cost you an hour or two.

Make sure that you always have keto-friendly foods on you. Invest in some food containers that you can easily put in your bag and take with you places. Keep them filled with things like nuts, vegetable sticks, yogurt dip and sliced avocados. At a sports game, in a meeting, out on a long shopping excursion, or anytime that you have to be away from home for more than a few hours, you can pop the containers out and recharge on ketogenic foods.

One challenge of the ketogenic diet is that many foods have to be eaten immediately after being prepared. The thought of eating scrambled eggs that have been in the refrigerator for a couple of days is less than appetizing. Look for recipes that can be prepared in advance and eaten throughout the week. Examples include curries, soups and casseroles. Take one day each week to prepare some dishes that can be refrigerated and eaten throughout the week. This will save you a lot of time and enable you to stay on track, even on your busiest days.

Know what local restaurants have keto-friendly options on their menus so that when you do go out to eat, you already know what you can order without derailing your diet. Just because something isn't labeled keto-friendly doesn't mean that it isn't. An omelet with cheese is probably fine, as long as you don't add hash browns or anything else on the side. If you are at a restaurant that doesn't have anything that appears to be keto-friendly, ask for something to be specially prepared, based on the ingredients that appear in the other foods on the menu. For example, if there are choices that contain avocados, cucumbers and oil and vinegar dressing, you can request that those ingredients be made into a salad.\

Take advantage of grocery delivery

Grocery shopping can be a time-consuming hassle, but nowadays, many stores offer grocery delivery. You select online what you want and when you want it to be delivered, then pay online via credit or debit card. This can shave hours every week off of the time you spend on maintaining your keto diet.

Keep in mind that grocery delivery usually carries a fee and may be more expensive than going to the store, so make sure that you are aware of the cost. If you live in a large city, there may be several different stores that offer grocery delivery that you can check out.

Let others know of your diet

Before going out with friends or going to visit relatives, let them know that you are on the ketogenic diet. Inform them that you don't expect them to prepare any special food for you but that there are many foods that you will not be able to eat. Try to select restaurants that you know have keto-friendly options so that you and your friends can enjoy eating whatever you prefer. And who knows? You may find that others want to join you on the ketogenic diet!

Make friends with others who are on the ketogenic diet

Joining a group of people who are already on the ketogenic diet can be a great way to achieve accountability with people who are working towards the same goals. People who have already been where you are can give you practical advice about how they dealt with the side effects of adjusting to the diet and a state of ketosis, as well as how to handle things like the holidays and those worried emails from your parents about the supposed dangers of going keto. They can also give you pointers about things like saving money on groceries and cooking keto meals separately from what your family normally eats.

While you should avoid preaching to your friends about going keto, some may see how much the diet has benefited you and want to join in. You can hook them up with your buddies who are already on the ketogenic diet and work together as accountability partners.

Exercise regularly

The benefits of exercise are so immense that it is a wonder that doctors don't prescribe it instead of medication. It boosts immunity, improves blood flow and circulation, elevates mood, increases metabolism, burns off the stress hormones that can accumulate after traumatic events or as part of a hectic daily life, burns calories, purges blood sugar, relieves constipation, reduces insulin, the list goes on and on. One reason nutritionists may be against the ketogenic diet is that it doesn't necessarily incorporate exercise.

Commonly, people get onto the ketogenic diet as a shortcut to losing weight instead of as part of a healthy lifestyle, which has to include exercise. If you go onto the ketogenic diet, it needs to be because you want to improve your health, not just because you want to lose weight. Losing weight is a side effect of increased health and wellness. You need to exercise for at least thirty minutes four times a week.

Going for a brisk walk in the evening or for a morning jog is a great way to get started with exercise. Taking the stairs instead of the elevator and parking further away from the store instead of fighting for a front-row parking spot are easy ways to incorporate exercise into your daily life. You may want to join a gym or buy in-home exercise equipment, but you don't have to. Most people who buy gym membership or exercise equipment never use it unless they were already exercising regularly beforehand.

The best way to make exercise a meaningful and regular part of your life is to make it enjoyable. Put on some music and listen to your favorite songs while you are running on the treadmill. Go for a walk with your family or a friend. You will soon find that you feel so much better, both physically and emotionally, that you will want to continue exercising as much as possible.

Plan keto nights with friends

Your friends and/or family don't understand the ketogenic diet and they frequently discourage you from following it. Your mom repeatedly sends you emails with articles about how dangerous the ketogenic diet is and your best friend keeps tempting you with your favorite carb-rich foods to try to get you to start eating "normally" again. They have no idea why you would spend so much time preparing high-fat meals at home. So show them!

Plan keto nights in which you prepare keto-friendly foods for your friends and family to try. Have all of the ingredients out and enlist their help to prepare the meal. They might find themselves pleasantly surprised at how appetizing the ketogenic diet really is and some might even decide to join you!

Drink lots of water

Because the water-rich foods that you probably once enjoyed, like mangoes and apples, are no longer staples in your diet, you are consuming significantly less water than before. Additionally, when you are first starting out on the ketogenic diet, your kidneys will have to work harder to process all of the fat you are consuming along with the glucose and glycogen stores that your body is burning through. You will have to be intentional about drinking a lot of water. You will probably need to drink one ounce for every pound of body weight. If you are 160 pounds, you will probably need 160 ounces of water per day.

Practice intermittent fasting

Intermittent fasting is the practice of fasting for between 16 and 48 hours at a time for the purpose of gaining health benefits. Intermittent fasting has numerous health benefits. It turns on your body's fat burning processes, improves mental clarity and gets you into a state of ketosis.

You naturally are going into a fasting state at night when you sleep, because you aren't eating. Intermittent fasting extends this state throughout the day. Some experts prescribe fasts as a prelude to beginning the ketogenic diet and others advise fasts as a way to get the most benefits out of it. This is actually much easier than you may think because the ketogenic diet leads to significantly less hunger. When fasting, make sure that you consume plenty of fluids. You may want to supplement with things like coconut oil and butter to help induce ketosis.

Decrease your stress levels

Many of us live hectic, stressful lives. We are busy from the time we wake up until we go to sleep and increasing demands are constantly placed on us. You may find that you are constantly stressed to please your boss at work, care for your children and/or aging parents, maintain your home, keep up with finances, the list goes on and on. Our use of smartphones keeps us constantly connected, which can easily mean that the boss expects us to be readily available to answer emails and phone calls after hours. With today's tough economy, you may find that you are working a lot of extra hours or even two jobs (or more!) to try to stay afloat financially. Just let it be said that stress is an epidemic and you are probably not immune to it.

The effects of stress can be disastrous for anyone's health. In response to stress, the body releases cortisol and adrenaline and induces a "fight or flight" response. Many people actually live in a perpetual fight-or-flight state and are unable to shut their minds down, even to be able to sleep at night. The cortisol causes fat to build up in the abdominal area, which is the most harmful place for fat to accumulate. Stress also causes blood pressure to rise and increases the risk of other heart diseases. It easily makes people irritable, causing harmful effects on their relationships. Mood disorders, like depression and anxiety, can develop. Chronic stress can also lead to autoimmune problems, digestive issues, insomnia, skin problems like eczema and acne, infertility and cognitive issues. It can also inhibit a state of ketosis because stress hormones actually raise blood sugar and insulin and drive down ketone production. Needless to say, reducing stress is an important step in maintaining a healthy lifestyle.

Think about what you can reasonably do to decrease the stress in your life. You may need to take major steps, like considering a job change or lowering your hours at work. You may need to make other small changes, like reducing your financial obligations or turning off your smartphone at certain hours. Many people find that working with a counselor to help them deal with the toxic effects of stress and identify its causes is very beneficial in improving their quality of life.

You may be going through a particularly stressful or even traumatic period in your life. If that is the case, maintaining a state of ketosis may not be a reasonable goal. Instead, aim to eat a low-carb, high-fat diet, exercise regularly and seek out support from family, friends and possibly a professional.

Monitor your health

Because the ketogenic diet induces so many chemical changes in your body's metabolism, you need to keep tabs on different markers of health. You can easily buy ketone-testing strips that measure your ketone production through breath, blood, or urine. The ketogenic diet tends to reduce the electrolytes in your body, so you may want to get a tool that measures electrolytes in order to ensure you have an adequate amount. Because the goal of the ketogenic diet is ultimately to suppress the use of glucose for energy by inducing ketosis, you may want to get some tools for testing your blood sugar and insulin levels. These tools are easily available, as they are frequently used by diabetics as part of their daily regimens.

There are easy ways to monitor whether or not you are dehydrated. If your urine is yellow, cloudy and/or has a strong odor, you are probably dehydrated and need to drink a lot of water. This can also mean that you are drinking enough fluids but not enough water, so cut back on things like milk, coffee and tea and replace them with water. Another dehydration test is to pinch your arm. If the skin immediately snaps back into place, you are fine. If it sags or takes a moment to return to its original position, then you are dehydrated.

If implemented correctly, the ketogenic diet can become a lifelong lifestyle of health and wellness that will improve your wellbeing for years to come.

Mistakes to Avoid

Now let's look at the top mistakes Keto Dieters make and strategies to overcome them. It is helpful to keep them in mind even after you are successfully leading a Keto Lifestyle.

Mistake 1: Not Knowing your Macro Proportions

Ketosis is a reversible phenomenon. So long as you are using fat as your primary food and burning ketones for energy you will be able to control your weight and blood sugar levels. As soon you switch back to carbs, eat too much of proteins or reduce the proportion of fat in your diet, the body goes back to burning sugar for energy.

That's why maintaining an optimum proportion of Fats, Proteins and Carbs in your diet is so important for a Ketogenic Diet. Majority of the people falter in keeping this balance of proportion in a sustainable way over a long period of time.

So what is the Optimum Proportion?

Again, the answer to this question is more nuanced than you would like to hear. In short, the answer is, Know Your Own Body. Please find the recommended ranges below, but you will have to work with your body to determine the optimum amounts suitable to keep you in Ketosis.

In terms of percentage ratio the following proportions are recommended:

- Fat 60-75%
- Protein 15-30%
- Carbs 5-10%

Broadly the proportion depends on the following factors:

- Your Body Mass Index
- Your Age
- Your Percentage Body Fat
- Your Activity Level

If you are just starting on your Keto Diet, it's best to restrict your carb intake to 20-30 grams per day (remember 1 big orange = 1 pint of beer = 20 grams carb). For a majority of people, carb intake range can be increased to 20-50 grams per day once you have achieved the desired weight loss and are in the weight maintenance phase. There are a number of Keto Calculator Apps you can find that will help you in calculating your exact macro proportions.

Mistake 2: Scale Watching

You need to accept the fact that being on a Keto Diet is a lifestyle change and not a crash diet. You will get there, keep calm and carry on!

It's natural for you to want to weigh yourself regularly to check progress when on a diet, but this is actually not a very accurate way to measure results. You need to realize that weight is just a number and is neither a very meaningful or accurate measure of how you are progressing nor an indicator of fat loss or physical fitness. Just remember that apart from your water weight that can fluctuate several pounds in a short span, the scale is a snapshot of what happened two weeks back.

What is the difference between your friend who weighs 300 lb. and an athlete who weighs the same? They do weigh the same but is their body composition the same?

It is important to understand that losing fat and weight are two different things. As we lose body fat and gain muscle mass especially for someone who has recently begun exercising, the scale would continue to show the same weight. Indicators that you are on track to losing weight even if the scale doesn't budge:

- Your tape measurements show a shrinking waistline.
- Your clothes are getting looser, you look slimmer and people around you notice the difference.
- You have lots of energy and want to exercise after living a sedentary lifestyle for years.
- Your health markers are improving.
- Your Body Mass Index (BMI) dips.
- Your mental focus improves, you don't experience afternoon slumps anymore.

Measure your Ketones

Measuring ketones is a good way to know that your body is in Ketosis and is burning the stored fat. There are a number of ways to measure ketones produced in your liver as your body goes through ketosis. These include urine test kits, blood test kits, breathalyzers and good old-fashioned observation techniques. Depending on your budget and interest, measuring ketones can be a good way to monitor results during ketogenic diet.

Mistake 3: Sugar Addiction

Sugar is the biggest hindrance to leading a healthy lifestyle. Removing sugar completely from your diet is absolutely necessary for a successful transition to Ketogenic Diet lifestyle. In fact, a gradual removal of this single substance from your diet alone will make you healthier than the majority of people. If you want to take one lesson from this book it is to completely remove sugar from your life.

The average per capita sugar consumption in America has risen to 153 grams per day from 9 grams per day back in 1822. Our bodies have got so used to sugar that in reality, it is difficult to get through a day without consuming sugar in some form. Being so readily available and ingrained in our lifestyle makes it all the more difficult to give up sweet foods. Check out the Resources section of the book for 56 different names of sugar used by the processed food industry to hide the amounts of added sugar in your food.

So what is Sugar? Sugar is simply Glucose + Fructose (The Sweet Part). It has:

- No healthy fats
- No protein
- No vitamins
- No enzymes

How Sugar makes us Eat More - Sugar triggers a chain reaction where high levels of sugar in the bloodstream results in increased insulin levels. This insulin, in turn, makes it difficult for the brain to receive the satiety signal. As a result, the brain is fooled to believe that the body is still hungry leading to excessive food consumption and weight gain.

How to Overcome Sugar Cravings:

- Reduce your Carb Intake: A high carb diet causes blood sugar to rise, which in turn signals the body to release insulin. You need to increase your consumption of protein and good fat to overcome this. Proteins are made up of amino acids, which are important for balancing hormones and sugar cravings. Healthy fats are a source of energy for our body and help reduce hunger pangs and provide satiety.

- Plan Your Meals in Advance: Hunger is not the best time to make rational decisions on what is best to eat. Planning ahead to include nutrient-rich food in your diet will help curb hunger swings and sugar cravings.
- L-Glutamine Dr. Julia Ross in her book "The Mood Curse" suggests that intense sugar cravings are due to stress, poor diet and deficiency of amino acids (to the extent that diet alone may not be able to correct it). She suggests a short-term supplementation of amino acid L- Glutamine.
- Check your Pantry: Keep sugary foods out of sight as much as possible.
- Watch Out for the Hidden Sugar: Low fat, sugar-free and diet foods contain added sugar or synthetic sweeteners in order to enhance the taste of the food and palatability. Get into the habit of going through the labeling for savory foods, juices, sauces, salad dressings and condiments. You will be surprised how many of them contain sugar.
- Avoid Artificial Sweeteners: Replacing sugar with a sugar substitute in the belief that it will reduce calorie intake and help in weight loss is a myth. Recent studies have shown that on the contrary artificial sweeteners

maintain the cravings for sweet food and increase appetite. Our body increases insulin secretion in anticipation that sugar will appear in the bloodstream. When the body doesn't receive the sugar, insulin uses the existing sugar in the bloodstream for energy. As a result, blood sugar levels drop and hunger increases leading to uncontrolled binging.

Mistake 4: Electrolyte Imbalance

Electrolytes are salts that flow in your bloodstream and carry an electric charge. They are essential for the cells in our body to function properly, whether it is to regulate blood pressure, help with muscle contraction or nervous system functions.

It is a well-known fact that on a Keto Diet the initial transition phase results in significant water loss. With the water are lost essential minerals like sodium and potassium, which triggers an electrolyte imbalance.

You will need about three times more electrolytes when on a Keto Diet as compared to a normal diet. Signs that you have an Electrolyte Imbalance:

- You are restless, have muscle aches, spasms and joint pains
- You have heart palpitations and find it difficult to sleep.
- You experience dizziness and fatigue I

Important Electrolytes Include:

<u>Sodium</u>

Responsible for maintaining fluid balance in our bodies, helps in muscle contraction and nerve signaling.

Sources of Sodium: Table Salt and Himalayan Pink Salt.

Magnesium:

One of the most under-appreciated minerals, Magnesium helps in maintaining a stable heart rate, bone building, the creation of DNA and RNA and normal nerve and muscle functions.

Sources of Magnesium: Almond, Salmon, Spices and Leafy Vegetables.

Potassium:

It aids muscle contraction, regulates heart contractions and keeps blood pressure stable. An imbalance of sodium and potassium is caused when we consume sodium-loaded processed foods and skip vegetables rich in potassium. This could lead to hypertension, heart attack and stroke.
Sources of Potassium: Avocado, Nuts and Dark Leafy Vegetables.

Calcium:

In addition to helping with the formation and maintenance of bones and teeth, calcium helps with cell division, cell clotting and transmission of nerve impulses.

Sources of Calcium: Almonds, Cheese and Broccoli.

Healthy individuals who are not working out extensively get their daily intake of electrolytes from the food they eat.

However, if you are sick, out on a very hot day or on a low carb diet, your electrolyte requirement spikes up.

Mistake 5: Fat Phobia

For years we have been told that eating fat will make you fat. Some of the most popular diets in the world are based on this premise. It is this social conditioning that leads us to subconsciously make choices that are low in fat.

As a result sugar and grains have been the primary source of the calories for most of us. Once you remove these two from your diet you will need to replace them with another energy source. If you don't you will feel hungry, tired and low all the time and will eventually switch back to carbs.

It is important to understand that there are two sources of energy – glucose and ketones. When on a low carb diet, sufficient intake of fat (60-75 % of total intake) leads us into ketosis and our body uses ketones for energy. However, if our body does not get into ketosis, it will look out for glucose for energy. It will either get it from carbohydrates or from protein (through Gluconeogenesis).

Keto Diet advocates a mix of saturated fats, omega 3s and monounsaturated fats.

Different types of Fat Present in our Food:

Saturated Fat (SFA):

They are stable fats, with long shelf life and suitable for high flame cooking. They help to keep in check your bone density, immune system and testosterone levels. Contrary to popular belief their consumption does not adversely affect the heart.

Sources of SFA: Meat, Egg, Butter, Ghee, Lard, Coconut Oil are good sources of Saturated Fat.

Monounsaturated Fat (MUFA):

They are liquid at room temperature and best for cold use for salads or after cooking. Good for the heart, they are now a popular choice of fat.

Sources of MUFA: Avocado, Olives and Nuts (especially macadamia).

Polyunsaturated Fat (PUFA):

This type of fats can be primarily divided into the naturally occurring Omega 3s and the industrially processed Omega 6 fats. PUFAs are unstable and fragile and not suitable for cooking. When heated, they react with oxygen to form harmful compounds called free radicals, which in turn raise our risk of heart diseases and cancer. Omega 3 consumption is good for our body but most of the PUFA cooking oil is high in omega 6, which is harmful.

The ideal ratio of Omega 6 to Omega 3 fats is 1: 1. However, in reality, the ratio is way higher than this, ranging from 10: 1 to 20: 1 on an average, so not only do we have a problem of excess Polyunsaturated fat, we also have a much higher proportion of omega 6 fats and deficiency of omega 3s.

Sources of healthy Omega 3s: Wild Salmon, Walnut, Fermented Cod Liver Oil, Macadamia Nuts and Grass-Fed Meat.

Trans Fat:

This is considered the worst form of fat and should be avoided. Trans fat is unsaturated fats primarily found in processed foods where through industrial process hydrogen is added to liquid vegetable oil to cause the fat to become solid at room temperature. This partially hydrogenated oil helps to increase the shelf life of processed food. It is linked to heart diseases and has an adverse effect on cholesterol levels.

Stay clear of products whose product label mentions words like "trans fat", "hydrogenated". It is worth noting that in the United States if per serving of any product anything lower than 0.5 grams then it can be labeled as 0 grams of trans fat. These hidden trans fats quickly add up if you consume multiple servings.

High-Fat Foods to Include in Your Diet:

- Avocados: Avocado, unlike most fruit, is loaded with monounsaturated fat oleic acid. This is the main fatty acid in olive oil and linked with various health benefits. It is a great source of potassium and fiber and helps lower triglyceride.
- Cheese: It is made from the milk of grass-fed animals is a good source of nutrients as it is high in saturated fats and omega 3-s, protein and amino acids
- Whole Eggs: Eggs are one of the most nutrient-dense foods and are loaded with vitamins and minerals.
- Fatty cuts of Meats and Fish: Include fatty cuts of grass-fed animals. Avoid chicken breasts or lean meat where the fat has been removed. Include fish like Salmon, Sardine, Mackerel and Trout in the meal plans. If you cannot eat fish then it is worth considering a supplement like Cod fish liver oil, which contains Omega 3-s and Vitamin D.

- Nuts: Nuts are loaded with Protein, Vitamin E and Magnesium in addition to healthy fats and are a great option to add to a meal when consumed in moderation. Almonds, Walnuts and Macadamia nuts are some of the healthy choices.
- Chia seeds: They are high in Omega 3 fatty acids and fiber. They can be a useful addition to your diet.
- Extra Virgin Olive Oil: Rich in vitamin E & K and loaded with antioxidants, extra virgin Olive oil is an excellent choice. The antioxidants in the oil help improve cardiovascular health, lower blood pressure, fight inflammation and protect LDL particles from oxidation in the blood.
- Coconut Oil: It contains 90% saturated fatty acids making it the richest source of saturated fat.
- Butter and Ghee (clarified butter): Butter has been demonized for long but Grass Fed butter is good for you. In addition to Vitamin A, E and K2 it contains Conjugated Linoleic Acid (CLA) and Butyrate. CLA helps in lowering fat percentage and Butyrate improves the gut and fights inflammation.
- Lard, Tallow and Bacon Fat from naturally raised animals are a great option for cooking and are high in healthy saturated and monounsaturated fats

Mistake 6: Carb-Loaded

So much has already been discussed about carbs. But I would like to reiterate that you should become aware of your carb tolerance. An athlete will probably have a greater carb tolerance than someone with a sedentary lifestyle. On the safer side, your carbs intake should not go beyond 20 grams max when you start your Keto Diet.

Getting rid of carbs may work in the short term, but there always comes a time when all of us start to crave for the starchy stuff. The temptation of having just that one small slice of bread can be overwhelming.

Let me warn you again though, Ketosis is a reversible state and can be broken very easily by just having that one small piece. Not only that, once you start eating that one piece, insulin level in your blood starts to rise which will play all kinds of havoc with you. Let me show you how a high carb diet affects us physiologically.

Why "Eat less and Exercise more" is Not a Solution: The conventional weight loss wisdom from the diet industry is 'Eat less and Exercise more'. This advice, derived from the calorie in calorie out (CICO) theory, falls flat in the world of complex human physiology. CICO completely ignores the inner workings of a human body and has led to lots of people abandoning their weight loss quest.

People who propagate CICO believe that Calorie IN = Calorie OUT + Stored Fat. So the amount of fat stored in the body depends upon the number of calories we consume minus the calories expended in bodily functions and exercise. Nothing can be far from the truth!

The human body has no way of measuring calories but has its own way of regulating fat. Insulin is the hormone that controls how much energy we expend and how much is stored as fat.

When we eat, the insulin goes up and the body starts storing fat. And eating equal calories of carb will raise insulin level more that eating equal calories of fat. That's why in human physiology; a calorie is not a calorie. As we stop eating, the insulin levels drop and the body stops storing fat. As the fasting continues body starts burning the stored fat.

That's why conventional (High Carb Low Fat) diets fail. Because of high insulin levels in carb-based diets, fat is being continuously stored. So even if you are eating lesser calories overall, insulin levels will remain high because of carb consumption and fat storage will continue. Ironically, weight gain continues and with increased appetite.

In a Low Carb High Fat (LCHF) diet, however, the insulin levels are lower. So when you consume equal calories of fat based food, a part of your energy needs will be met with the stored body fat. So using an LCHF diet for fat loss is more effective as your appetite is decreasing with a steady decline in body fat.

Mistake 7: Excessive Drinking

Keto Diet does not mean the end of your social life. Sure hit the bars, but you have to do so responsibly. Please remember if it tastes sweet, it's probably sugary and should be avoided.

You will have to keep a check on what you drink and how much you drink. Beer and wine should be especially avoided as they contain a lot of carbs and sugar. When you drink, your body will metabolize it on priority before other sources of energy, as it cannot store alcohol. This means that although alcohol consumption will not completely throw you out of ketosis it will for sure prolong the timeline for your goals as when the body is burning alcohol for energy it is unable to metabolize the stored fat.

Remember to drink plenty of water in between your drinks. Keto lowers your alcohol tolerance level so keep sufficient gap between drinks.

Mistake 8: Importance of Proteins

Like many of us do you also have the notion that Ketogenic Diet is all about keeping your carbs low and increasing your fat intake?

For a lot of people just keeping low on carbs, helps in weight loss. However, some people are more metabolically resistant than others and despite keeping their carb levels below 20 grams per day continue to gain weight. It is in such cases worth looking at your protein intake.

We give little attention to how much protein we need to consume in order to stay in ketosis. Our body cannot make protein on its own and as such protein is an important macronutrient without which your body wouldn't be able to carry out the necessary tissue building and repair functions.

What is Gluconeogenesis?

It is worth understanding the process of gluconeogenesis here. It is a metabolic process by which our body produces glucose from non-carbohydrate sources – amino acids in the protein being one of them.

Gluconeogenesis is an essential process without which we probably cannot survive for long, especially if we need to go without food, as our body needs a constant and steady flow of glucose to keep the brain and red blood cells functioning.

When we consume more protein than our body needs the excess is turned into glucose. This glucose is over and above the minimum requirement of the body and results in weight gain.

Optimum Protein Intake:

There are various theories on how you can calculate the ideal protein intake taking your weight in pounds and then multiply it by 0.6 and 1.0. This will then give you the ideal range for your protein intake in grams.

An easier way is to pick a level of protein and while still keeping carbs below 20 grams monitor how you are doing for that quantity of protein intake. If you continue to struggle, keep shifting your intake downwards until you hit the sweet spot.

It is worth noting that when you are experimenting to find your ideal level of protein intake you must keep your carbs low and have adequate monounsaturated and saturated fats to give you the much-needed satiety.

If you are struggling with weight loss due to being more sensitive to proteins, try and avoid leaner cuts of meat like chicken breast as that would elevate your blood sugar levels and make you gain weight just by having too much protein than your body needs. On the other side, cuts of meats with saturated fat will automatically lower your protein intake and help in weight loss.

Mistake 9: Falling for Fake Products

Wouldn't it be great if we could eat bread, pasta and chocolate and still lose weight rapidly without hunger or all the complicated diseases associated with sugar?

There are plenty of shady businesses that promise the impossible. An excellent example is low carb pasta from Dreamfields that tastes like any regular pasta. They are even made from regular starchy wheat, but the manufacturer still claims that our body does not absorb the carbs as their pasta is protected from some "patent pending process".

The problem is that their claims are completely bogus and raises blood sugar like any regular pasta. Based on several types of research it was proved that their pasta behaved like regular pasta and Dreamfields had to pay a settlement fine of $ 8 million because they had lied; however, by then they had sold their fake low carb pasta for 10 years.

There are many similar examples of fake products. Carbzone is a company that claims to sell low carb products. They claim their tortilla made from whole wheat is low carb; however, on testing it showed to contain 3 times as many carbs as stated on the label. Even low carb chocolate cookies from the Atkins Company often contain sugar alcohol like Maltitol, which the maker pretends to not raise blood sugar. However, this claim has no merit and about half of it does end up raising blood sugar. The manufactures omit sugar alcohols from the net carb count so that they can market it as low carb.

In short, do not fall for fake products. If it tastes like bread, pasta or chocolate then the reality is that it is bread, pasta and chocolate.

Lifestyle Problems

Now, let's look at the lifestyle challenges that some followers may face. We will also look at the best ways that these can be addressed.

Keto on a Budget

Some people worry about following Ketogenic Diet on a budget. But actually, once you start, you'll find that your monthly spend on food will actually go down. The reasons for the same are mentioned below:
1. You will buy fresh base ingredients instead of processed ingredients
2. Once you hit ketosis, you will observe that satiety comes much earlier and you will eat less. This is another sign that you are in the state of Ketosis.

Farmer's market is a great place to shop for fresh ingredients while on Keto. You will find pocket-friendly bargains

there while supporting the local community. Moreover, you will learn more about your food by being in direct touch with the producers.

Eating Out

Eating in a restaurant can seem daunting when you first start following a ketogenic diet. Actually, it doesn't need to be difficult if you follow a few simple rules.

Try to stick to meat, dairy, or vegetable dishes that don't come with rice, pasta, or bread. Things like steak with salad are a good choice, as are salads on their own with cheese or meat added. Other good choices when eating out can be fish or seafood with non-starchy vegetables.

Just be careful to have them with olive oil rather than dressings, which can be high in sugar. Also remember that it is up to you if you want to customize your order and ask for things like sauces to be left out, so don't be afraid to ask! It also is worth checking with the restaurants if they have Keto/ Paleo/ LCHF friendly dishes.

Eating with Friends and Family

Friends and family may not understand Ketogenic Diet and may want you to eat whatever they are eating, especially if you have done so in the past. At the end of the day, you may not be able to explain the principles of Ketogenic Diet to them in a way that changes their minds, but just remember that it is up to you to choose what to eat. They may just be convinced when they see your weight loss and renewed energy levels!

Conclusion

The keto diet can be hard to maintain which is why you should try to get into it slowly. The first step is to slowly transition yourself into it instead of just pushing your body to the limit. So, don't abandon all the food that you used to eat, instead cut them out of your diet slowly.

The second step is to jump right into it and wait for the benefits to start showing. Now, it might happen that the diet isn't working for you, but you shouldn't worry about that. Our bodies are different which is why not all diets can work for everyone. You should consult your doctor if you are not losing any weight even after following the diet for a long time.

Lastly, remember to stay motivated and tell yourself why you're doing this. It can be hard to cut out all the carbs from your life, but you can always use some simple techniques to keep yourself motived. You should take pictures of yourself after every few months and notice the progress you are making, this will help you to stay on track.

Finally, if you enjoyed this book, then I'd like to ask you for a favor, would you be kind enough to leave a review for this book on Amazon? It'd be greatly appreciated!

Thank you and good luck!

Preview Of Intermittent fasting: **Beginners Guide To Weight Loss For Men And Women With Intermittent Fasting**

Do you want a diet that will help you lose weight and improve your overall health? Do you want a diet that doesn't prescribe calorie counting? It does sound quite wonderful if you can achieve your weight loss and health goals without counting calories, doesn't it? If your answer is yes, then you are in for a pleasant surprise! Intermittent Fasting is the diet that you have been looking for. Fasting is not a new concept and has been around for a long time. Intermittent Fasting is a simple variation of fasting and is very helpful. This dieting protocol alternates between periods of fasting and eating.

In this book, you will learn about the basics of Intermittent Fasting, the changes that take place in your body, the benefits it offers, different methods of Intermittent Fasting, tips to exercise, common FAQs and much more. Intermittent Fasting is quite simple. You merely need to make a couple of changes to your eating habits and you are good to go.

If you are fascinated by this diet and want to learn more about it, then let us start right now!

Chapter One:
History of Intermittent Fasting

Unlike other forms of conventional dieting, the concept of fasting is quite unambiguous and easy to understand. Did you know that most of us tend to unconsciously follow the protocols of Intermittent Fasting? Do you ever skip having breakfast or dinner? If you do, then you are following an Intermittent Fasting protocol. You will learn about the different methods of Intermittent Fasting in the coming chapters.

Our hunter and gatherer caveman ancestors had to seek food in nature. So, they were often on a fast until they found some nourishment. Then agriculture was introduced, and it led to the formation of human civilization. Whenever there was food scarcity or whenever the seasons changed, fasting was the norm. They used to maintain stocks of grain and meat in cities and castles for harsh winters. Before the introduction of agriculture, shortage of rainfall meant a spell of famine and people used to fast to make their food supplies last longer. Enough rain was quintessential to meet the grain requirement.

Along with civilizations, there came religions. Religions grew when people were living in close quarters and shared similar beliefs. Most of the religions prescribe fasting. Hinduism refers to fasting as Vaasa, and Hindus observe it during festivals or other auspicious days. Fasting is also considered to be a form of penance. Islam prescribes fasting during the holy month of Ramzan. A similar practice is present in Judaism and is known as Yom Kippur. There's a period of fasting before Easter in the Catholic faith.

Technology and innovations play a vital role in the evolution of humans. Industrialization revolutionized the food industry. Mass production of food products meant that the markets were constantly flooded with food products. Apart from this, the way humans view and consume food has also undergone a major change. The human body didn't get a chance to sufficiently adapt itself to the rampant changes brought about by industrialization and agriculture. All this meant that a host of health problems soon followed. Intermittent Fasting is quite an old practice. Even though it is an old practice, humans have just begun to understand and truly appreciate the various benefits this diet offers. Whenever you fast, you give your body a chance to cleanse itself - not just cleanse but even repair and regenerate itself from within.

Essentially, while fasting your body gets to burn out all the excess fat it has stored. Human beings have evolved in such a manner that we can fast without any health risks and that is normal. Body fat is the reserve of food that the body has stashed away for a rainy day. If you don't consume food, your body will simply reach into this reserve to provide you with energy. There needs to be balance in everything you do. There's a yin and a yang. The same rule applies to eating and fasting as well. Fasting is the flip side of eating. If you aren't eating, then you are fasting. When you eat something, this leads to an accumulation of food energy that isn't going to be made use of immediately. A portion of this is stored away. A hormone known as insulin is responsible for storing the food energy. When you eat something, there is a spike in the level of insulin. This facilitates the storage of energy in two different ways. Sugars are linked into long chains and this is known as glycogen. The rest is stored in the liver. When the space available has been maxed out, the liver starts turning the rest into fat. Some of this fat so created is stored in the liver and the rest is stored in the form of fat cells in the rest of your body. There isn't a limit on fat creation. So, there are two forms of energy stores in our bodies. One is easily accessible and has a limited storage space (glycogen), and the other is the harder to reach energy without a limit on storage (body fat).

This process is essentially reversed when you don't eat, that is during fasting. There will be a reduction in the level of insulin and this enables your body to reach into its storage of fat cells and burn this to provide energy. The most easily attainable source of energy for your body is glycogen. This is broken down into molecules of glucose that sustains your body. This can provide sufficient energy for your body to function for 24 hours or longer. After this, your body will reach into its fat reserves to generate energy. Your body will do this only while feeding or fasting. Either your body will be storing energy, or it will be burning energy. Only either of these processes can take place at any given time. If there is a balance between eating and fasting, then there will not be any weight gain. Over a period of time, you will start gaining weight if you haven't given your body sufficient time to burn all the food it has stored. To restore balance, you will need to give your body sufficient time to burn the food energy. This can be accomplished by fasting. This is how our bodies are designed. Intermittent Fasting helps to restore this much-needed balance.

Circadian Rhythm and Intermittent Fasting

Human beings, like other organisms, have a biological circadian clock that ensures that the physiological processes in the body are performed at the right time. The circadian rhythm is on all day long and it affects the biology and the behavior of humans. Any disruption in this rhythm has a negative effect on the metabolism and it can cause several metabolic dysfunctions like obesity, diabetes and a host of cardiovascular diseases. The primary factor that affects the circadian rhythm is the signal to eat. It is responsible for metabolic, physiological and behavioral pathways in the body. All these pathways are responsible for making sure that your body performs optimally. Apart from this, they also ensure that your body is healthy. You can use behavioral intervention to regulate the body's circadian rhythm. Yes, you guessed it right! Intermittent Fasting is a means of behavioral intervention that will streamline the circadian rhythm. This in turn leads to better gene expression and improvement in your body's health and metabolism.

Gut Microbiome and Intermittent Fasting

The gastrointestinal tract regulates multiple processes within your body. In other words, your gut helps regulate different physiological and biochemical functions in your body. For instance, the metabolic reaction to glucose and the blood flow are higher during the day than at night. Even a small fluctuation in the circadian rhythm can impair your metabolism and increases the risk of several chronic diseases. The microbiome present in the gut is usually referred to as the second brain. It is known as the second brain because of the influence it has over your metabolism and physiology. Intermittent Fasting has a positive impact on the gut microbiome. It makes the gut less permeable, reduces the chances of systemic inflammation and improves overall energy balance.

Lifestyle Behavior and Intermittent Fasting

Intermittent Fasting helps change different health-related behaviors like calorie consumption, energy expenditure and your sleep cycle. Therefore, it is not a surprise that these are the three primary functions that help fight the most significant health concern that plagues the human community, obesity. You will learn more about the different benefits it offers in the coming chapters.

Chapter Two:
Different Methods of Fasting

Intermittent Fasting is a varied and a dynamic diet that offers multiple health benefits. There are different methods of Intermittent Fasting that you can follow, and you need to select one that will meet your needs. So, read on to learn more about the different methods of Intermittent Fasting.

16/8 Method

If you follow this method of Intermittent Fasting, you must fast for 16 hours daily. If you fast for 16 hours, the eating window comes down to 8 hours. You can squeeze in two or three healthy meals within this time frame. It is popularly known as the LeanGains method. The creator of this variant of Intermittent Fasting was Martin Berkhan, a fitness expert. This method can be something as simple as skipping your breakfast and directly having your first meal at noon and your last one at about 8 p.m.

The next meal you can have will be on the following day at noon. So, you will fast for 16 hours and, frankly, you will not even feel like you were fasting for 16 hours. Ideally, women must not fast for more than 14 hours. If you like to wake up early and eat breakfast, then have a hearty breakfast, then you need to make sure that your last meal is at around 4 or 6 in the evening.

You are free to consume all sorts of calorie-free beverages throughout the day like water, black coffee or any other herbal teas. You need to make sure that you don't include any sugar in your drinks, since it will effectively break your fast. If you want to lose weight, then you must not binge on junk foods when you break your fast. This method works, only if you strictly follow the protocols of the diet.

The 5:2 Diet

In this variation of the diet, you need to restrict your calorie intake on two days of the week and eat like you normally do on the other days. On the days you need to restrict your calorie intake, the calories you consume must be between 500 and 600. Michael Mosley is the creator of this diet and it is also known as the Fast diet. On the days that you fast, you must ensure you don't consume more than 600 calories. You can squeeze in two small meals within this calorie limit. This diet is ideal for all those who don't like the idea of fasting daily.

Eat-stop-Eat

In this form of Intermittent Fasting, you must fast for 24 hours, once or twice in a week. Brad Pilon, a famous fitness expert, created this diet.

You can choose the days you want to fast on. For instance, if your fast starts at 8 p.m. on Monday night, then you will break your fast only at 8 p.m. on Tuesday night. You can decide when you want to fast, if you fast for 24-hours. You cannot consume any solid food during your fasting period but can have calorie-free beverages. You must ensure that you are consuming healthy meals on the normal days. If you are just getting started with fasting, then this might be a little complicated. Instead, it is a good idea to start with either of the previous methods and then make your way toward this dieting protocol. If you want to follow this diet, then you need self-discipline and self-control.

Make sure that your fasting period never exceeds 48 hours. So, don't try to fast on two days continuously and pace it evenly.

Alternate Day Fasting

If you want to follow this method of Intermittent Fasting, then you need to consume 500 calories on every alternate day. If you are not a fan of a strict diet, then this will work well for you. You can eat like you normally do on all days except for the ones with the calorie restriction.

Warrior Diet

Ori Hofmekler, a famous fitness expert, was the creator of this diet. In this method, you need to have small portions of raw fruits and vegetables during the day and end your day with a hearty meal at night. You will essentially be fasting throughout the day and will feast at night. The eating window in this method is restricted to about 4 hours. The food that you can consume on this diet is quite like the food you can consume while following a Paleo diet. So, you are free to fill up on foods that are unprocessed. It essentially means that you can eat only those foods that our cavemen ancestors had access to. If you feel like your caveman ancestors could not have eaten something, then neither can you. If you don't want to fast all day long, you can snack on fruit and vegetables. It will keep your hunger pangs at bay.

Spontaneous Fasting

As the name suggests, you merely need to skip meals spontaneously. There is no fixed plan. If you don't feel like eating, you simply need to skip a meal. There will be times when you don't have time to eat or when you don't feel like eating. So, whenever you skip a meal, you are effectively following the protocols of this diet. It will not do your body any harm if you skip meals from time to time.

Chapter Three:
Benefits of Intermittent Fasting

Perhaps the most common reason why people opt for Intermittent Fasting is to lose weight. Apart from weight loss, there are various other benefits this diet offers, and you will learn about them in this chapter.

Weight loss

Intermittent Fasting alternates between periods of eating and fasting. If you fast, naturally your calorie intake will reduce, and it also helps you maintain your weight loss. It also prevents you from indulging in mindless eating. Whenever you eat something, your body converts the food into glucose and fat. It uses the glucose immediately and stores the fat for later use. When you skip a few meals, your body starts to reach into its internal stores of fat to provide energy. As soon as your body starts burning fats due to the shortage of glucose, you will start to lose weight. Also, most of the fat that you lose is from the abdominal region. If you want a flat tummy, then this is the perfect diet for you.

Sleep

Lack of sleep is a primary cause of obesity. When your body doesn't get enough sleep, the internal mechanism of burning fat suffers. Intermittent Fasting regulates your sleep cycle and, in turn, it makes your body effectively burn fats. A good sleep cycle has different physiological benefits - it makes you feel energetic and elevates your overall mood.

Resistance to illnesses

Intermittent Fasting helps in the growth and the regeneration of cells. Did you know that the human body has an internal mechanism that helps repair damaged cells? Intermittent Fasting helps kickstart this mechanism. It improves the overall functioning of all the cells in the body. So, it is directly responsible for improving your body's natural defense mechanism by increasing its resistance to diseases and illnesses.

A healthy heart

Intermittent Fasting assists in weight loss, and weight loss improves your cardiovascular health. A buildup of plaque in blood vessels is known as atherosclerosis. This is the primary cause for various cardiovascular diseases. Endothelium is the thin lining of blood vessels and any dysfunction in it results in atherosclerosis. Obesity is the primary problem that plagues humanity and is also the main reason for the increase of plaque deposits in the blood vessels. Stress and inflammation also increase the severity of this problem. Intermittent Fasting tackles the buildup of fat and helps tackle obesity. So, all you need to do is follow the simple protocols of Intermittent Fasting to improve your overall health.

A healthy gut

There are several millions of microorganisms present in your digestive system. These microorganisms help improve the overall functioning of your digestive system and are known as gut microbiome. Intermittent

Fasting improves the health of these microbiome and improves your digestive health. A healthy digestive system helps in better absorption of food and improves the functioning of your stomach.

Tackles diabetes

Diabetes is a serious problem on its own. It is also a primary indicator of the increase in risk factors of various cardiovascular diseases like heart attacks and strokes. When the glucose level increases alarmingly in the bloodstream and there isn't enough insulin to process this glucose, it causes diabetes. When the body is resistant to insulin, it becomes difficult to regulate the insulin levels in the body. Intermittent Fasting reduces insulin sensitivity and helps tackle diabetes.

Reduces inflammation

Whenever your body feels there is an internal problem, its natural defense is inflammation. It doesn't mean that all forms of inflammation are desirable. Inflammation can cause several serious health conditions like arthritis, atherosclerosis and other neurodegenerative disorders.

Any inflammation of this nature is known as chronic inflammation and is quite painful. Chronic inflammation can restrict your body's movements too. If you want to keep inflammation in check, then Intermittent Fasting will certainly come in handy.

Promotes cell repair

When you fast, the cells in your body start the process of waste removal. Waste removal means the breaking down of all dysfunctional cells and proteins and is known as autophagy. Autophagy offers protection against several degenerative diseases like Alzheimer's and cancer. You don't like accumulating garbage in your home, do you?

Similarly, your body must not hold onto any unnecessary toxins. Autophagy is the body's way of getting rid of all things unnecessary.

Chapter Four:
What to Avoid During a Fast

Intermittent Fasting helps rectify and reverse several health conditions, but it doesn't mean that it is ideal for everyone. An important thing that you need to keep in mind is that you need to consult your medical practitioner before you start this diet.

Who can fast?

The following people can fast

Healthy adults

All healthy adults can fast. It helps cleanse the body and there aren't any reasons why a healthy adult cannot fast.

Children

Usually, it isn't suitable for children up to the age of 18 to fast; however, children can fast. A child must only fast for a short duration and must not fast for prolonged periods. A perfectly healthy child doesn't have to fast. The general exception to this rule is all those who suffer from obesity. A child needs plenty of nutrition for growth and their body needs nourishment constantly. If the child is less than 18 years, please consult a medical practitioner.

Type-2 diabetes

Fasting helps reverse the harmful effects of type-2 diabetes. If you suffer from this, then you are free to fast. Before you start any diet, you must always consult your medical practitioner.

Who Cannot Fast?
Pregnant women

As such, there is no conclusive proof that shows the effect of Intermittent Fasting on a fetus. It is better to abstain from any diets if you are pregnant or are trying to conceive. If you are planning to start a family, then your body needs plenty of nutrition and you must not restrict your diet at this point of time. Also, mothers who are breast-feeding need to abstain from Intermittent Fasting. Fasting reduces the nutrition available in breast milk and it also affects the quantity of milk that is produced.

Any medical conditions

If you have any health concerns related to the kidney or the liver, then you must not fast. You need to consult a doctor before you fast if you have any pre-existing medical conditions. If you use any medication for high blood pressure or have a weak immune system, then you must not fast. You can fast even if you have medical conditions, but don't forget to consult your doctor.

If you have recently had a major surgery, then please abstain from fasting. Also, fasting is not ideal for all those who are recovering from any major illness.

Eating disorders

If you have any eating disorders or are recovering from an eating disorder, then you must not fast. Fasting can cause a relapse and you need to avoid it at any cost.

Afraid to fast

If fasting scares you, then don't fast. Fear is an unnecessary stressor and it will just cause problems. Fear is a powerful emotion and can alter your psychological makeup. If you think you cannot handle fasting, then don't try to fast. If you want this diet to generate positive results, you need to have an open mindset!

Foods to Avoid and Eat

When you are following the protocols of Intermittent Fasting, the primary focus is not on what you eat, but it is on when you eat. Just because it doesn't focus on what you eat, it doesn't mean that you stuff yourself with carbs and sugar-laden treats. For best results, it is a good idea to stay away from all processed foods and opt for healthy foods. It means that it is a good idea to avoid all sugary treats or at least try to limit them as much as you possibly can. So, avoid cookies, chocolates, cakes, and all packaged sweets.

Stay away from foods rich in unhealthy fats and carbs like burgers, pizzas and all fast foods. Say no to foods that are devoid of all protein and are full of sugars and carbs. Avoid soy products if you want to lose weight. Soy products are rich in estrogen and a high level of estrogen will not do you any good.

You need to maintain a calorie deficit if you want to lose weight. The higher the level of insulin in your body, the less fat you will lose. Carbs and sugars increase the level of insulin. So, if you want to regulate your insulin levels, you need to avoid carbs.

There are some people who believe that you can eat a lot of protein, fruit and vegetables while fasting. If you eat all this during a fast, you aren't effectively fasting, are you? Even if you had a couple of drops of honey to your morning tea, you will be effectively breaking your fast. Just because you aren't permitted to eat anything, doesn't mean that you stop drinking water.

Your body needs at least 8 glasses of water to stay hydrated and ensure that you are thoroughly hydrated. Drinking water will make you feel fuller and helps you to avoid any hunger pangs.

You are free to consume all calorie-free beverages like black tea, black coffee, green tea, herbal teas and carbonated water. Try to limit your caffeine intake. Caffeine has a diuretic effect on the body and too much of it can cause dehydration due to the loss of electrolytes. Try to limit your caffeine intake to about two cups of coffee or any other caffeinated calorie-free drink of your choice. It might seem quite tempting to add some sugar or cream to your coffee, or perhaps some honey to your tea. If you do this, you will cause a spike in your insulin levels. When there is a spike in your insulin levels, your body stops burning fat and it negates the benefits of fasting. You must try to avoid anything that will cause a spike in your insulin levels and effectively break your fast. Some people believe that chewing sugar-free gum will keep hunger at bay. Even all those products that are labeled as "no sugar" or "sugar-free" include some carbs in them.

If you really want to lose weight and want to improve your overall health, then it is a good idea to stay away from all forms of alcoholic drinks as well.

Alcohol contains a lot of carbs that can sneak up on you unknowingly. Intermittent Fasting helps cleanse your body. So, if you really want to cleanse your body then you need to avoid all the things that will result in the internal buildup of toxins. So, stay away from alcohol to improve the efficiency of this diet.

Natural Remedies

Table of Contents

Introduction 1

1-Hypertension 2

2-Hyperlipidemia (elevated cholesterol) 4

3-Diabetes 6

4-Arthritis 8

5-Anxiety 10

6-Asthma 11

7-Hypothyroidism 13

8-Cellulite 15

10-Urinary Tract Infection (UTI) 20

11-Constipation 23

13-Eczema 26

14-Erectile Dysfunction & Impotence 28

15-Dandruff 30

16-Migraine Headaches 32

17-Breast Cancer 34

18-Ovarian Cysts 36

19-Brittle Nails 38

20-Irritable Bowel Syndrome (IBS) 40

Conclusion: 42

Introduction

Let's face it, we don't need pharmaceuticals to be healthy. When given the proper nutritional support, the body can heal itself without the need for toxic and expensive medicine. That's not to say that all conventional medicine is without value but rather that there are alternative remedies that should be explored first and for long enough to give the body a fighting chance.

In this guide, I have selected some of my favorite remedies for common conditions that most Americans have suffered or know someone who has suffered with. These cures are practical and affordable and more than likely, contain items that can easily be picked up from a grocery or local health food store.

1-Hypertension

As being one of the most common conditions affecting both men and women, hypertension or high blood pressure is said to affect more than 70 million American adults and that number is rapidly growing. Typical medical treatments for this condition include prescription medication such as beta-blockers and ACE inhibitor drugs both of which are dangerous and with prolonged use, can lead to problems in other areas of the body. Although these drugs are effective in treating the condition, they do not address the underlying problem.

In addition to prescribing drugs, Doctors urge patients to limit the amount salt in their diet. This has been one of the biggest theories in relation to hypertension yet there just is not enough evidence to prove it. In fact, numerous studies have proven time after time that a salt restricted diet does not help to cure hypertension.

So what is the best remedy for high blood pressure?

Calcium and lots of it! Foods high in calcium may help but must be used in conjunction with supplements.

Also, in order for calcium to work effectively, adding vitamin D and Magnesium can help.

Numerous theories conclude that calcium helps to keep the body alkaline by preventing the body's pH level from becoming acidic. This works because hypertension cannot be prevalent in an alkaline body.

What other natural cures can you use for hypertension?

Baking Soda. Yes, you read that correctly. Baking soda is easily one of the fastest most affordable ways to lower hypertension naturally. Best of all, you probably already have a box laying around somewhere in your pantry since it is such a common kitchen item.

Baking soda is an excellent way to boost your pH levels quickly and efficiently. It's important to monitor your body's pH levels regularly to ensure that this method is working for you and to help measure the difference. An easy way to do this is to pick up alkaline test strips which can detect and measure the body's pH levels through urine.

How to take:

Mix 1/8 teaspoon of baking soda in 1 cup of water and add 2 tbsp. of apple cider vinegar and take twice daily. This should be repeated for approximately two weeks. After that, take only the apple cider vinegar and water alone for another two weeks. Once the two weeks are up, you may resume adding the baking soda. Continue this two weeks on and off cycle with the baking soda until you begin to see an improvement in your symptoms.

Since this is a safe and natural method, it can be continued for as long as you wish as long as you follow the directions above.

Potassium which is found in a number of common foods is known to essentially "clean out" artery walls and flush excess sodium from the body. One of the best sources of potassium is liquid organic or unpasteurized apple cider vinegar which contains beneficial microorganisms and enzymes also known as the "Mother" apple.

2-Hyperlipidemia (elevated cholesterol)

If your recent blood work showed that you have elevated cholesterol and triglyceride levels, chances are, there is an underlying problem that needs addressing first. Taking cholesterol lowering drugs will only serve to treat the symptom but will not help to fix the cause of the problem.

There are a few common myths surrounding cholesterol that are pushed on the general public by health care providers and the pharmaceutical industry.

First Myth: The lower the cholesterol is in your body, the healthier you are. This could not be further from the truth. Cholesterol is essential to your health and overall well-being. In fact, the only time it becomes problematic is when there is an excess of it. Simply put, we cannot live without cholesterol. The "safe range" for this essential nutrient was once thought to be around 400 (4.0). Today, the "safe range" is below 200 (2.0). Despite this, death from heart disease has actually increased dramatically in the last 30 years and is expected to increase in years to come.

You're probably thinking, how does this make sense? Cholesterol is crucial to the proper functioning of the nervous system and liver as well as a crucial building block for adrenal and sex hormones. What's more, only 10% of one's daily need comes from the human body. The rest must be supplied through ones diet.

Second Myth: Animal products high in cholesterol such as full fat milk products, eggs, and red meat, are bad for you. This theory has never been proven and in fact, numerous studies have disproven its credibility.

An Eskimos diet consists of 70% animal fat, meat, and cholesterol. Despite this, a research study conducted on Eskimo health proved that their cholesterol and triglyceride levels were found to be low and that their risks for heart disease, stroke, and cancer were even lower.

As far as eggs go, study after study has shown that eggs do not raise cholesterol levels. In fact, they have been said to lower cholesterol since they contain lecithin (which is known to naturally reduce cholesterol). So, let's through this myth out once and for all!

What about butter? This is another horrid myth perpetuated by the pharmaceutical industry. It appears that the real culprit is processed oils and margarine. Butter in and of itself is not proven to raise cholesterol. In fact, countries like Sweden and Denmark who are the biggest consumers of butter have shown to have normal cholesterol levels. So go ahead and spread some on your toast today!

Third Myth: High cholesterol is a disease caused by heredity. Ladies and gentleman, this is a pure theory that has never been proven to be true. Do not fall for this.

High cholesterol is caused primarily by an individual's diet and standard of living such as excessive alcohol consumption, smoking, nutrient imbalance, and having a sedentary lifestyle.

Now that we've discussed the myths, let's discuss what you can do if you have been diagnosed with high cholesterol.

Fish oil supplement: I know, this one is pushed on us a lot...but there is a lot of evidence to back it up. Fish oil has been proven time after time to lower cholesterol and triglyceride levels. Consuming dark meat/cold water fish on a frequent basis can be just what you need. However, if you're not a big fan of fish, taking a good quality Omega-3 Supplement can be comparable.

Foods to incorporate into your diet to naturally lower cholesterol:

- **Oats:** bring triglyceride levels down fast due to the fiber it contains.
- **Apples:** Opt for organic apples whenever possible—any kind will do.
- **Avocados**: contain healthy mono-saturated fats, including oleic acid which has been shown to lower cholesterol.
- **Dark greens:** Spinach, broccoli, and lettuce to be specific. Try organic whenever possible.
- **Lecithin:** This can be purchased in supplemental form or is found in egg yolks.
- **Blueberries:** containing powerful antioxidants, bioflavonoids, and vitamin C, these little gems play a huge role in disease prevention overall.
- **Soy:** Aim for organic whenever possible. Soy will help to activate enzymes within the body to help reduce cholesterol.
- **Flax Seeds:** these can be added to a smoothie or sprinkled on your salad or cereal.
- **Garlic:** Helps to enhance the immune system and lower cholesterol and blood pressure levels.
- **Water:** aim for at least 2 liters of water per day for optimal results.

3-Diabetes

Over the last 10 years alone, the number of people diagnosed with diabetes has skyrocketed. It is now estimated that 25.8 million adults and children have this nasty disease. Left untreated, diabetes can potentially lead to a wide range of health risks including coma and death.

So what causes diabetes and what are some of the symptoms associated with it?

Normally, the body's metabolic process consists of converting carbohydrates into a sugar called glucose. This then circulates in a person's bloodstream and signals the pancreas to secrete a hormone called insulin. This is the hormone that initiates the body's cells to absorb the glucose.

Once the glucose is absorbed by the cell, it becomes fuel to help generate energy or gets stored as fat in the body. In a person who has diabetes, this delicate process is disrupted. Instead, the pancreas releases little to no insulin or the body's cells reject the insulin. This causes the cells to be starved of glucose leading to a wide variety of symptoms such as weakness, fatigue, and frequent urination. Symptoms range from mild to more severe symptoms such as labored breathing, trembling, dizziness, and in worst cases, loss of consciousness.

There are 2 types of diabetes mellitus and they are type I and type II. Type I develops in childhood years due to minimal or no insulin production by the pancreas. Type I diabetics are required to take synthetic insulin to help keep their glucose levels lowered.

Type II diabetes which is also known as adult-onsite diabetes is the most common making up 90-95% of all diabetics. In the case of type II diabetes, the pancreas over-produces insulin but it is not absorbed by the cells so it is left to circulate in the bloodstream until it is flushed out in urine. Constantly elevated levels of blood glucose poses serious health risks.

So, what can you do about Diabetes?

Besides exercising regularly and eating fresh organic fruits and veggies, there are a few different natural remedies you can try at home to help manage and eventually eliminate diabetes. Please keep in mind that you should never stop taking your diabetes medication or insulin without consulting with your doctor first. You should continue to monitor your insulin regularly until a plan of action has been established and started under the guidance of your health care provider.

Coconut Oil. Yum! This miracle food has been known to treat a wide variety of illnesses and diabetes is definitely one of them. Best of all, it tastes great too. By consuming at least 3-4 tbsp. of coconut oil per day, you can successfully treat and reverse type II diabetes.

Coconut oil helps to reduce the constant sugar and carbohydrate cravings in individuals with diabetes. This helps to better control the body's blood sugar levels and keep them within normal range. Also, since most diabetics are also overweight, the coconut oil can also help with weight loss which in turn can help to manage diabetes better.

Black seeds: Nature's wonder seeds! Black seeds are an anti-inflammatory and immune system booster treating a score of illnesses which includes diabetes. A recent study showed that just 2 grams of black seeds a day helped to reduce fasting glucose levels, decrease insulin resistance, and increase cell function in diabetic participants.

The easiest way to take black seeds is to purchase the oil which can be found online or at most health food stores. For dosage information, refer to the directions contained on the bottle.

Green Tea can also be used to treat diabetes. It contains powerful polyphenol antioxidants which are well-known for increasing insulin sensitivity and stabilizing blood glucose levels.

Be sure to drink 4-6 cups a day for diabetes. Green tea supplements can be used instead if you cannot stomach the bitterness from the tea.

4-Arthritis

There are many natural remedies for arthritis that modern medical doctors fail to address. Unfortunately, this incredibility debilitating disease continues to affect millions of people worldwide.

Besides not being able to do the things they once were able to do, arthritis sufferers and their loved ones are severely misinformed about the types of natural treatments that are available to them. Most conventional medical treatments only focus on treating the symptoms of arthritis and fail to address the underlying problem.

Arthritis is an extremely profitable disease and the pharmaceutical industry is not interested in educating the masses on non-conventional treatments. Drug induced therapy appears to be the number one standard medical treatment available to patients for treating their arthritis. In the long run however, most of these medications are further damaging joints and overall health.

What's more, these drugs begin to lose their effectiveness over time requiring the need to switch medication and or increase the dosage. In addition, the medication can increase the risk for various illnesses such as heart attack, liver and kidney malfunction, and hypertension. The side effects associated with these medications can include depression, insomnia, and mood swings to name a few.

In addition to medication, surgery is oftentimes suggested by doctors to treat arthritis however this is a risky procedure that can cause serious complications.

So what can be done?

Baking soda and apple cider vinegar...yes again! This powerful combination is one of the most incredible ways to remedy arthritis naturally. I have tried this one personally and can vouch for it 100% (at least for me).

I mentioned some of the benefits of baking soda earlier but to recap, baking soda helps to elevate your body's pH levels. This helps to alkalize the body and keep it in a healthy state and since disease cannot live in an alkalized body, you should start to see relief immediately. It's crucial to keep in mind that you should not consume more than 2 tsp of baking soda a day to stay within the safe zone.

Apple cider vinegar is truly a powerful natural antibiotic which helps to heal the gut and destroy pathogens. In addition, it helps to replenish the digestive track with probiotics so that no bad bacteria can mess with your internal system! Pretty great if you ask me.

How to make remedy

Mix 2 tbsps. of apple cider vinegar with ½ teaspoon of baking soda in 1 cup of water. Add a teaspoon of black strap molasses or honey for extra benefit and taste. Drink twice daily and then gradually increase to three times daily. This can be done for 3 weeks and then the baking soda can be discontinued. You can continue to drink apple cider vinegar daily for as long as you want after that.

What else?

Turmeric & Ginger Tea. Both of these amazing ingredients are powerful anti-inflammatories which will help with the pain and swelling associated with arthritis. Turmeric contains a strong antioxidant that helps to lower the levels of two enzymes that are responsible for causing inflammation.

Here's how to take:

Combine 2 cups of water with a 1 teaspoon of ground turmeric, 1 teaspoon of ground ginger, and add honey to sweeten. Boil 2 cups of water and add the turmeric and ginger. Let simmer and then stand for 10 minutes. Finally, go ahead and strain it, add honey and enjoy! This can be enjoyed twice a day for as long as you'd like or until the pain is gone.

Blackstrap Molasses is a black syrup substance which is a by-product made by through the refining of sugar beets or sugarcane into sugar using a boiling process. Unlike regular sugar, molasses is rich in vitamins and minerals such as magnesium, calcium and potassium making it a potent home remedy for arthritis. Due to the nutrients contained within it, molasses helps to regulate the function of muscles and nerves and helps to make bones stronger.

Here's how to take:

This one is easy. Heat one cup of water until warm (not hot). Add 1 tbsp. of blackstrap molasses stir until dissolved.
Drink one cup daily.

5-Anxiety

Anxiety and stress are unfortunately rampant in our society today and we all experience them on occasion. Anxiety is a natural response to stress or fear which alerts us to a perceived danger or threat. Without it, human beings would have no way of anticipating and adequately preparing for, an adverse situation ahead of them.

Anxiety only becomes problematic if it begins to affect ones daily life. This can easily spiral into a condition called Generalized Anxiety Disorder which is characterized by marked excessive worry regarding ordinary things. If you are like the millions of people around the world who suffer with this, understand that there are many natural remedies available for treatment.

Since anxiety produces many distressing physical symptoms such as a pounding heart, sweating, dizziness, and shortness of breath, it can cause added worry associated with the fear of death. The secret to treating these physical symptoms is to first calm the body and mind. A calm body will always lead to a calm mind and vice versa.

The good news is that there are many different home remedies you can use to alleviate anxiety and help calm your body down.

Celery. Stay with me now...Celery is high in folic acid and potassium. Deficiencies with either of these can cause nervousness. Consume approximately 2 cups of celery either raw or cooked with your meals for 2 weeks or until symptoms begin to subside.

Rosemary: This popular spice has a calming effect on the nerves simply by inhaling the aroma. To enhance the benefits, burn a sprig or purchase rosemary oil and simply breathe in the aroma.

A tea can also be made from Rosemary to help ward off anxiety but adding 2 teaspoons of dried rosemary to 1 cup of boiling water. Let stand for 10 minutes and then drink.

Orange. Who doesn't love a nice tall glass of OJ with their breakfast in the morning? Did you know it can also help with anxiety-induced tachycardia (racing heart). Simply mix 1 teaspoon of honey and a pinch of nutmeg into 1 cup of orange juice and drink.

Also, like the rosemary mentioned above, the aroma of orange has been known to reduce anxiety and its symptoms. You can inhale orange by simply peeling a fresh orange or boiling orange peels and simply breathing in the steam.

6-Asthma

Asthma is a chronic illness which involves the airways in the lungs which are responsible for allowing air to flow in and out of the lungs. Asthma occurs when this delicate process is disrupted due to inflammation of the airways causing the muscles around the airways to tighten making it difficult to breathe. Symptoms associated with is condition include shortness of breath, tightness in chest, coughing, and wheezing.

Over the last few years alone, reported cases of asthma have risen dramatically. It is now estimated that today, close to 34 million Americans have been diagnosed with asthma. In addition, according to the CDC, asthma costs upwards of 56 million dollars a year in medical costs, lost school and work days, and early deaths and this number is continuing to grow.

So what is the cause of this rampant growth of cases?

The theory that asthma is genetically inherited is just that, a theory! Therefore, there are other causes responsible for the incredible spike in asthma rates. Here are a few:

- **Increase in pollutants** which is found in our air, water, and food. Unfortunately, there is no way to eliminate these pollutants entirely but you can limit your exposure by cutting down on chemicals from the diet.
- **Decreased immunity in children and adults:** This should go without saying but when your immune system is compromised, your risks of contracting illnesses such as asthma increases. Therefore, you need to address the underlying problem by making sure you're taking care of your immune system.
- **Increased use of asthma medications:** Regular use of these medications can lead to an exacerbation in symptoms. This is because they negatively affect the immune system by causing a disruption to the body's endocrine system.

Is there anything you can do besides taking dangerous medication? Of course!

Hydrogren Peroxide Inhalation Therapy can be a very powerful natural remedy for asthma. Most people have this sitting in their medicine cabinet at home making it a very practical and affordable treatment. Best of all, it can work within minutes.

Here's the method:

1. Start by purchasing 3% food grade Hydrogren Peroxide and a nasal pump containing a generic nasal decongestant (you'll be dumping it out so the cheaper the better)
2. After emptying out the contents of the pump, make sure to sterilize the bottle properly using hot water and soap making sure all soap is properly rinsed out.
3. Fill the empty bottle with the peroxide and while pointing at the back of the throat, inhale and pump the spray 5-6 times (while inhaling). **Make sure that you are NOT inhaling it up the nose.

This method can be repeated 5 times a day or every 3 hours or so and can be used for as long as needed.

Another great home remedy is, **Ginger.** Due to it's anti-inflammatory components, this is actually one of the most effective herbs for helping to treat asthma symptoms. Ginger helps to relax and smoothen muscle tissue in the airways and can help to dissolve phlegm. Not to mention, it's excellent at boosting the immune system due to the powerful vitamins and minerals contained within it.

How to take?

The best way to enjoy ginger is by pouring boiling hot water on a few slices of ginger and letting it steep for 20 minutes before sipping. Add honey if desired. This can be enjoyed 2-3 times per day for as long as you'd like or until symptoms have decreased.

Home relief for asthma can also be achieved through consuming garlic.

World renowned for its antiviral properties, garlic is an excellent anti-inflammatory food item that can be used for asthma. Garlic can easily be classified as "nature's antibiotic" as it can clear congestion in the nose, throat, and lungs and help to fight infections that typically trigger asthma attacks. Simply eat 1-2 cloves a day or use a garlic capsule to gain the most benefits.

7-Hypothyroidism

Hypothyroidism is the term that is used to describe an underactive thyroid gland. This is when the thyroid gland cannot keep up with normal hormone production to keep the body running normally. Common causes associated with this condition are autoimmune disease, radiation treatment, and the surgical removal of the thyroid.

Luckily, this condition is very easy to cure using simple remedies and treatments. Although there isn't a single cure that exists for hypothyroidism, relief can take place after an individual has modified his/her lifestyle and has incorporated vital supplements.

Traditional methods of treating hypothyroidism include modern day medicine and hormone therapy. Both of these methods can be harmful and even fatal especially when used in the long term.

Luckily, there are safer, more effective ways to treat this condition. Most of which the pharmaceutical industries will try and refute since it means zero profit for them. One way is to incorporate a healthy, well-balanced diet free from chemicals and processed sugar and rich in fruits, vegetables, and whole grains. In addition, it is also important to begin exercising on a frequent basis—even if it means just walking, get up and get moving.

Let's look at a few additional home remedies to try for hypothyroidism.

Apples, Pears, and Peaches. All are an excellent source of fiber which helps to keep you regular. This in turn helps to regulate hormones as well! All three of these fruits help to calm hormone imbalances in a woman's body helping her relax. They work best when combined.
Here is a wonderful juice recipe to try:

Combine 1-apple, 1-pear, and 2-peaches. Blend together and pour through a strainer to remove pulp if needed. This can be drank once daily for as long as you'd like or until signs and symptoms subside.

Vitamin D: This is best when derived from natural sunlight. It's important to get at least 30-minutes of natural sunlight exposure daily. Put away the sunblock and sunglasses during that time and really allow the sun to penetrate your skin and eyes. Allowing the sunlight to be absorbed adequately, helps to stimulate the body's pineal and pituitary glands. These glands are responsible for releasing T_3 & R_4 hormones which helps to speed up the body's metabolism. This can help lead to weight loss and a dramatic increase in energy.

If natural sunlight isn't an option for you, you can also purchase a high potency vitamin D3 and fish oil supplement to ensure that you receive a minimum of 2000 IU per day.

Flaxseeds are rich in plant omega-3s and help to produce a hormone-like substance which is called prostaglandins. This in turn helps to stimulate thyroid hormone production which helps to prevent and treat hypothyroidism.

8-Cellulite

This is a very well-known problem that millions of women (and some men) around the world suffer with. Cellulite basically describes normal fat beneath the skin which appears bumpy due to pushing against connective tissue. Although not a serious problem, it is certainly not desired and can be cosmetically unpleasant.

Each year, billions of dollars are spent for reducing the appearance of cellulite. Treatment options include cellulite reduction creams and surgical invasive and non-invasive procedures. Fortunately, there are more practical and affordable options available which need to be sought out and practiced regularly in order to remove cellulite for good!

It's estimated that 85% of women suffer from cellulite in the United States. It can affect women of all ages, shapes, and sizes which means that essentially anyone can have it. The most common areas of the body that are affected include the buttocks, thighs, back of legs, hips, and stomach.

What causes Cellulite?

There are many factors that can lead to the development of cellulite. The most common causes include hormonal changes as well as toxic buildup of chemicals in the fat cells. In addition, cellulite can be caused by an unhealthy diet, dehydration, poor circulation, and a sedentary lifestyle.

So what are some natural home remedies you can use to treat this embarrassing condition?

Cayenne pepper. There is very little that this amazing spice cannot do. It can absolutely help with weight loss and cellulite since it helps to increase circulation and blood flow. In addition, it is well known for being a strong detoxifier as well.

How to take:

You can easily incorporate 1 teaspoon of cayenne pepper in your cooking twice a day or more. Or you can prepare this drink:

- Add 1 tsp cayenne pepper
- 1 tsp of finely grated ginger
- Juice from 1 lemon
- 1 cup of warm water

Mix ingredients together and drink twice daily. This can be used for as long as you wish or until cellulite begins to disappear. Keep in mind that this needs to be incorporated with a healthy diet to help maximize your results. What else?

Apple cider vinegar. Yes, again. This stuff really is the cure to everything isn't it? Apple cider vinegar contains essential minerals which help in detoxifying the body and removing excess fluid retention. This in turn helps to reduce the appearance of cellulite and if used for long enough, will help to remove it all together!

This remedy can be used both internally and externally. For external use, mix equal parts of apple cider vinegar and water and rub on the affected area. Wrap area in plastic wrap and place a warm compress on top (towel works best) before you take a shower. For internal use, mix 2 tbsp. of apple cider vinegar in a glass of water and drink before each meal. This can be done 3 times per day and can be repeated for as long as you'd like or until symptoms begin to subside.

Water, water, water. This one seems like a no-brainer but many people do not associate being adequately hydrated with cellulite reduction. The truth is, water DOES help in reducing the appearance of cellulite by giving skin a healthy glow and smoothing the surface. In addition, since it helps with detoxification as well, you can maximize your results by making sure to drink at least 8 glasses per day.

9-Multiple Sclerosis

Multiple Sclerosis (MS) is an erratic and often debilitating disease that affects the central nervous system disrupting the natural flow of information between the brain and the body. MS is classified as an auto-immune disorder in which the immune system mistakenly turns on the body and begins to attack the cells including the myelin sheath—the insulation material surrounding nerve fibers. As time passes, this insulation gets damaged and can negatively impact the communication process between the brain, nerves, and other parts of the body.

Symptoms associated with this disease can vary dramatically from person to person however, the most common include; numbness, loss of vision, tremors or shaking, vertigo, muscle weakness, depression, speech problems, fatigue, and cognitive problems.

Standard treatment for this devastating disease are even more distressing. Toxic pharmaceutical drugs and steroids are typically prescribed costing upwards of $30,000 a year on medication alone. What's alarming is that these drugs are not designed to cure MS but rather treat symptoms only and slow the overall progression of the disease. As usual, drugs fails to address the underlying issue at hand.

So what can we do right now to reverse this condition?

Ginger, Cayenne, Cinnamon, and Turmeric. What do all of these spices have in common? They are all potent anti-inflammatory foods which help to boost the immune system. Since inflammation is basically the a key factor in the development of neurodegeneration diseases such as multiple sclerosis, incorporating these spices in your everyday diet can be largely beneficial in the long run as they will help to alkalize the body.

Turmeric in particular has been used to treat a variety of ailments including toothache, menstrual difficulties, jaundice, and even flatulence. This miracle spice can be consumed either fresh or in powdered form.

Here is a wonderful drink recipe to try using Turmeric

- 2 cups of almond or coconut milk
- 1 tsp of raw honey
- 1 tsp of Turmeric
- ½ tsp of Cinnamon
- ¼ tsp ginger powder or small piece of ginger (peeled)

1. Blend all ingredients and pour into small sauce pan
2. Cook for 5 minutes until hot (not boiling) and drink immediately

What else?

Calcium & Magnesium. Both are crucial elements for the stability and development of the myelin sheath. Calcium helps with communication between the body and brain via the nerve signals while magnesium assists in the muscle contraction and relaxation. Aside from trying to incorporate more foods with these 2 essential nutrients, a good idea would be to get a strong calcium and magnesium supplement.

An excellent way to absorb magnesium, is through the skin. This can be achieved by spraying magnesium directly on the skin. Symptoms have been said to decrease in as little as 2 weeks after starting this regimen. It should be noted thought that this can cause some skin irritation in the interim—a pretty small price to pay for big long term relief. You can purchase a pre-mixed spray or for half the price, you can make your own.

Here's how:

- ½ cup of Magnesium Chloride Flakes
- ½ cup of distilled water
- Glass Bowl
- Spray bottle

Directions:

1. Boil distilled water and pour into bowl
2. Add magnesium chloride flakes and stir until the flakes are completely dissolved
3. Let the mixture cool and then pour in spray bottle

This can then be sprayed on the body (legs, arms, and stomach), once or twice a day aiming for about 15 sprays per area. Leave on for about an hour prior to washing off.

What about the types of food to eat? Are there any that are better than others? The answer is yes!

Fresh fruit and vegetables: Make sure to consume raw for maximum benefit. Seek out fruits and veggies that contain lecithin-a substance found in plants (and animal products) that helps to strength the nerves. Veggies that contain this ingredient include cabbage and bean sprouts. Of course, green veggies which are high in folic acid and B-vitamins are an excellent choice as well.

Eggs-surprise? Eggs are an incredible source of powerful nutrients and contain healthy fats which help support your brain and nervous system. For best results, aim to have at least 2 servings a day.

Fish: Cold water fish to be precise such as salmon, tuna, mackerel, herring, and my personal favorite, sardines. Aim for 3 servings per week if at all possible. Of course, if you cannot stomach fish—a supplement can be substituted.

Try and incorporate these foods/supplements into your diet and be prepared to see improvement. Of course, make sure to buy all organic when possible and try to incorporate exercise into your routine as well.

10-Urinary Tract Infection (UTI)

The urinary tract system is responsible for expelling waste and excess water from the body. It is comprised of the bladder, kidneys, ureters and the urethra. The kidneys are responsible for filtering and removing waste from the blood and forming urine which then travels down the ureters into the bladder until it is removed through the process of urination through the urethra.

Urinary tract infections have become widespread and common in our western countries. In fact, it ranks as second only to the common cold. The numbers of diagnosed cases are staggering and are said to be somewhere around 10 million per year. Needless to say, millions of dollars are spent yearly on treatments and doctors' visits and a great majority of patients are women. This is due to the biological structure of the urethra in women as it is shorter.

Symptoms of a urinary tract infection are not fun and can include (among many other symptoms) burning while urinating, frequent urge to urinate, and pain in the lower abdomen. If the problem isn't treated, the infection could spread to the kidneys leading to kidney damage. Symptoms of a kidney infection can be quiet severe and include fever, and pain in the lower abdomen and back. It's important to seek medical attention if you believe you have this infection.

Most people head to their doctors for treatment and are prescribed antibiotics. The problem with this however is that although they may be treating the symptoms in the short term, antibiotics rarely kill the microbes causing the UTI. In addition, they are killing the good bacteria in the digestive track which in turn, leads to the growth of bad bacteria. This can then lead to recurring infection within the urinary tract as well as release toxins into the bloodstream.

So what can be done naturally?

Cranberries. Sure, you've more than likely heard of this remedy but do you know why? Cranberries have been used to treat urinary tract infections for many years due to their high concentration of a substance called proanthocyanins. This helps to stop bacteria from clinging to the walls of the urinary tract. The urine is then able to essentially wash away the bacteria. In addition, cranberries are extremely high in a substance called D-Mannose. This has been studied for several years for its ability to attract bacteria helping it bind to it and then flushing it out of system during urination.

It was once recommended to simply eat cranberries or drink cranberry juice. After numerous studies however, this method has shown to be less effective than once thought. The reasoning behind this is that one must consume a large number of cranberries in order to achieve relief. Also, because most cranberry juice is high in sugar, it may have a reverse effect and cause bacteria to multiply further.

> A more effective alternative is to take a cranberry supplement instead such as a D-Mannose supplement.

This can have excellent results—and work quickly, since it contains a very concentrated amount of the compound.

This supplement should be taken for a few days (1 tablet 4 times per day) until the UTI symptoms have cleared up.

Let's look at which foods can help:

Blueberries: These amazing little gems are nature's perfect food. Rich in essential antioxidants, blueberries are known for optimizing human healthy by helping to combat free radicals that can wreak havoc on cellular structures and DNA. In addition, blueberries are an excellent natural remedy for UTI. In fact, they bear a striking resemblance to cranberries in that they contain the similar bacteria-inhibiting properties. Try and consume them raw and organic when possible.

Pineapples. My personal favorite. They contain bromelain which is an enzyme that is known for being a fantastic cure for UTI. It is also rich in vitamin C which not only helps to strengthen the immune system, but can also keep the bladder running efficiently.

Last but not least…

Probiotics! You can take a supplement for this, or try eating fermented foods such as yogurt, kefir, kambucha, and sauerkraut. Probiotics help to balance out the good bacteria in your gut—and everyone knows that a healthy gut=healthy overall body! This includes healing the bacterial infection within the bladder.

Here is a recipe for sauerkraut:
- 4 heads of shredded green or red cabbage
- ¼ cup of salt

1. Place cabbage in a mason jar and pound it to release the moisture making sure to sprinkle it with salt.
2. Keep the mixture below the top by about 1 inch to take expansion into account. You may need to add more in this step and make sure that the water extracted during the pounding process is enough to entire cover the cabbage. If not, mix 1 tbs of salt to 3 cups of water and add to jar.
3. Press the cabbage and keep under the brine putting pressure on the top using a weighted item such as a rock.

4. Place the jar in a warm area within the kitchen and allow it to ferment for 7-10 days. Keep it covered with a clean towel to keep bugs and dust out.
5. Make sure to remove any mold that forms at the surface and keep the cabbage immersed in the brine.
6. Once you are satisfied with the taste, place in refrigerator.

...And that's it! Easy peasy. This can be enjoyed alone or paired with your favorite foods (my favorite is brisket).

11-Constipation

This dreaded ailment affects the lives of millions of Americans each day. In a perfect world, one would have a bowel movement 3 times per day to ensure optimal colon health. However, bowel movement frequency varies among people. Some find themselves going 2 times a day while others only go about 3 times per week. This can be normal in and of itself. However, if one is experiencing uncomfortable bloating, and passing stool that is rock solid or large in size, it is highly likely that they're suffering from constipation. Anytime your stool is delayed by days or even over a week, and then accompanied by painful hard stool, natural relief should be sought out.

Being constipated means that the colon is not functioning optimally. This can cause unhealthy bacteria and parasites to grow and multiply. In addition, toxic liquids can then be recirculated into the body as they are not getting expelled properly causing a plethora of additional health problems.

So what causes constipation?

Although there are many causes of constipation, a poor diet is almost always the number one cause. This is because overly processed and refined foods are not digested as easily as natural healthy foods and therefore, are harder to eliminate. In addition, lack of fiber and an adequate consumption of water can both lead to constipation.

There are however many other causes for constipation. They include:

- Medical conditions such as IBS, cancer, MS, and hypothyroidism
- Stress and Anxiety
- Lack of physical activity
- Certain types of medication
- Over consumption of dairy products
- Artificial sweeteners

Let's take a look at some natural home remedies:

Salt Cleanse. What's great about salt is that it adds water into the bowel causing stools to soften up. This makes going to the bathroom a lot easier and more comfortable. Baking soda can be used as well as it has a similar effect. Both can be used together for a more severe case of constipation.

Directions for Salt cleanse

Mix 2-3 tsp of either salt or baking soda in cup of warm water and drink. This can be repeated every 4 hours until the bowels move. Keep in mind that frequently drinking fresh filtered water on a regular basis (at least 8 glasses per day) can help to naturally prevent constipation.

What else helps?

Olive oil. This is definitely a tried and true method of beating constipation. What's great about it is that most people have olive oil laying around in their pantry anyway and it's safe and natural to use—making it perfect for long-term use. Olive oil provides multiple benefits one of which is its ability to encourage the gallbladder to stimulate more bile which is a natural laxative.

What's more, its texture and consistency helps to lubricate the digestive system helping to move things through nicely. Rich in vitamins E and K and high in Omega 3 and 6 fatty acids, Olive oil can reinforce the health of your digestive track and when taken on a regular basis, can prevent constipation all together.

How to take?

Mix 1 tbsp. of extra virgin olive oil with 1 tsp of lemon juice and swallow. Repeat this once daily preferably before bed. Adding lemon can make taking the olive oil a little more bearable not to mention, lemon is also said to aid in constipation as well due to its high acidity. As stated earlier, this can be a long-term solution to prevent constipation but can also be used in the short term until symptoms are cleared. Remember to always buy extra virgin kind that is 100% olive oil.

Let's take a look at what else can help.

Black strap molasses. This dark, syrupy-like substance, provides a multitude of benefits and is rich in vitamins and minerals. What's more, it has a laxative effect in that it helps ensure regular bowel movements. In addition, it has high levels of magnesium and since constipation can arise due to a magnesium deficiency.

The best way to get relief is to mix 2 tbsp. of blackstrap molasses to ½ cup of warm water three times per day to help with constipation. Take preferably before bed.

12-Greying hair

This is a problem we all face at some point in our lives and in most cases, there are no proven ways to treat or reverse grey hair especially when it is age related. However, premature greying of the hair can be treated and reversed. The best way to achieve this is to begin both internal and external treatments.

Since grey hair can be caused by a mineral deficiency, it's important to begin taking a mineral supplement. The best way to do this is by purchasing a good **colloidal mineral** supplement. Since colloidal minerals have all of the minerals the body needs, and is provided in a easy-to-absorb form, it makes it a great choice for fighting greys.

In addition to this, a good quality **colloidal copper** can be added to the regimen as well. This makes for an excellent topical external treatment as well—simply dab some of the liquid colloidal copper to the scalp and massage.

Although internal treatments are extremely important and to be used as the first step in reversing greys, external remedies can be utilized as well:

Lemon and onion juice. Ok, it doesn't sound very appealing, I know. But, this can be a very powerful remedy which has been used for several centuries in successfully curing grey hair—long before the inventions of hair dyes. Simply slice an onion and rub on scalp pressing firmly as you go to help release the juices. Follow up by squeezing some lemon all over and begin massaging. If you can get past the smell, go ahead and continue this treatment daily for best results.

13-Eczema

That "itch you can't scratch" feeling that eczema brings, is not only uncomfortable but can often times be painful as well. Not to mention, eczema can be cosmetically unappealing as severe cases can cause discolored or blistering of the skin. Eczema is the general term used to describe a non-contagious inflammation of the skin that results in dryness and redness in the skin as well as unbearable itchiness. Excessive scratching of the skin, can further aggravate the condition and lead to broken or bleeding skin.

There are varying types of eczema but the most common form is Atopic Eczema. This form is more common in children and can be triggered by a several factors including allergens, skin irritants, bacteria & viruses, temperature, food, and stress. Individuals living in urban areas and dry climates seem to be more prone to this condition and although children seem to be more susceptible, it can reappear during adult years as well.

Once the cause is identified and treated, symptoms of eczema can clear up on their own. It's important to take a look at the composition of the skin first before researching a solution. Our skin is comprised of the epidermis which is the outer layer and the dermis which is the second layer. The epidermis is composed of cells filled with fat and water; a healthy epidermis is rich in moisture because of these 2 elements.

The oils in the skin help with enhancing the skins ability to retain water. In individuals with eczema, this delicate balance is disrupted as the skin begins producing less fats than normal. This causes the gaps between cells to widen leading to an eventual loss of water and moisture from the dermis. This explains why certain types of soaps can make eczema worse by stripping away the lipids produced by the skin leading to dryness and cracked skin.

So what types of home remedies can work to correct the problem?

Coconut oil. We learned earlier that coconut oil has many wonderful benefits and can be used to treat conditions such as diabetes. It also has wonderful topical benefits as well and does an excellent job of penetrating the skin and filling out the space in between the cells and restoring moisture.

How to apply: rinse area with water and pat dry. Then, take a generous amount of coconut oil and rub into skin. This can be reapplied during the day as needed.

Let's look at what else works:

Make your own body-butter. It's much easier than it sounds, trust me! A good quality body butter can really be an effective treatment for soothing inflamed skin. This can be made using Shea butter, Coconut oil, Jojoba, and Beeswax.

Shea butter's amazing benefits come from its fatty acid compound which gives it an ability to repair and soften damaged skin. In addition, its properties help to reduce inflammation making it an excellent choice in fighting eczema. Beeswax is to be used simply for thickening this butter as well as protecting and softening the skin. Jojoba isn't an actual oil but a liquid wax and mimics the same oils found in our skin. Combined together with the amazing healing power of coconut oil, and you have yourself quite the treatment!

Here's how to use this remedy

Gather the following items:

- 2 tbsp. shea butter
- 2 tbsp. beeswax
- 6 tbsp. Coconut oil
- 4 tbsp. essential oil of your choice
- Glass jar

Directions:

Melt jojoba and beeswax in a double boiler. Stir in coconut oil until combined and lower the heat. Begin adding the shea butter stirring vigorously as it melts. When complete, pour in airtight jar and add a few drops of the essential oil. Allow mixture to cool and apply to affected areas as needed.

Let's look at a final remedy:

Cornstarch and oil. Yes, you probably have a canister of this in your pantry now…so go and get it. Cornstarch mixed with oil can be an excellent paste to help soothe the skin. Simply add equal parts cornstarch and oil of your choice (I recommend grapeseed or olive oil) and mix together until a spreadable paste forms. Be mindful that the paste is not too thick or thin. This can be left on the skin for 20-30 minutes and then rinsed with water.

14-Erectile Dysfunction & Impotence

Erectile dysfunction or impotence refers to the incapacity to achieve or sustain an erection sufficient enough for sexual intercourse. Although this can occur to men at any age, it is the most common among men who are over the age of 50.

Many people who suffer with this condition can feel down and alone in their struggles. Truth is however, erectile dysfunction is actually a quite common problem to have. In fact, it is estimated that more than half of the male population suffer from impotence (According to the Cleveland Clinic).

Often times, this problem goes untreated since most men find it difficult to open up and admit that they have trouble attaining and sustaining an erection. Many men even find it difficult to talk about it with their partner since sexual performance is such as strong indication of masculinity.

Let's start with addressing the causes:

Erectile dysfunction in and of itself, is not an actual disease but rather a symptom of another problem within your body. Some common causes include but are not limited to: diabetes, high cholesterol, prostate disease, hypertension, and depression. In addition to these possible causes, the two underlying factors associated with E.D. and also related to many of these aforementioned conditions are low testosterone and poor blood circulation. Coupling this with pharmaceutical drugs is a recipe for disaster as many of them can lead to additional problems down the line.

The good news however is that there are natural remedies that can treat E.D. easily and effectively. Let's take a look.

Watermelon. Your favorite summer fruit just got sweeter. Watermelon juice contains citrulline which is an amino acid that is said to improve blood flow to the penis. This one is simple, simply juice watermelon and drink the juice directly, or just eat it whole.

Cayenne Pepper & Garlic can be a powerful combination in treating E.D. This is because, cayenne pepper helps to increase circulation throughout the body and this includes the genital area. In addition, garlic helps with blood flow by dilating the blood vessels. Try incorporating them both into your cooking and if desired, try them in capsule form. These can be taken 3 times a day after each meal. Keep in mind that the cayenne pepper can aggravate the lining of stomach when taken without food.

Apple Cider Vinegar. You're not surprised, I'm sure. We've already taken a look at some of the wonderful benefits of this miracle food item. It can be beneficial to almost every ailment known to man and erectile dysfunction is no exception. The good news is that it goes to work within a couple of hours of consuming and usually only requires a couple of doses.

Although Apple Cider Vinegar doesn't treat E.D. directly, it helps to treat the underlying problems that are said to cause it such as the ones mentioned earlier. It also repairs blood vessels and nerve fibers within the penis and reduces pain and inflammation of the prostate gland. So give it a shot!

15-Dandruff

Dandruff is simply a chronic condition marked by flaking of the skin on the scalp. Not only is it common, but dandruff is rarely serious and isn't contagious at all. Aside from being an embarrassing problem, many people find it rather difficult to treat as most traditional methods aim at treating the symptoms only. It's important first to pinpoint the underlying causes of this condition.

Dandruff is the result of a dry scalp or a skin condition known as seborrheic dermatitis. In addition, other causes include eczema, psoriasis and more commonly, a yeast-like fungus called malassezia. This is a normal fungus which is present on normal, healthy scalps and only becomes a problem when it begins to grow excessively. This can cause the scalp to get irritated and begin shedding dead skin cells at a rapid rate.

Oil on the scalp then combines with the dead skin resulting in clumps known as "dandruff flakes". I know, it doesn't sound very appetizing. To make matters worse, individuals suffering with dandruff often times have very oily hair as well. The good news is that dandruff including severe cases, can be treated and controlled naturally.

Baking Soda. This one is up there with ACV as being extremely versatile and effective at treating a multitude of ailments including dandruff.

The best way to use this natural treatment for dandruff is to wet the hair and rub a handful of it vigorously into the scalp before washing off. Baking soda reduces the overactive fungi and leaves your hair soft and flake free. Although this method can dry the hair out at first, when used for a minimum of 2-weeks, successful results can be achieved as you begin to notice your scalp producing natural oils.

Olive Oil. This one happens to be my personal favorite as I always have a bottle or two of it in my kitchen! Olive oil is chock full of antioxidants and vitamins E and A which improve scalp/hair health by providing nourishment and reversing heat damage. What's more is that it contains antibacterial and anti-fungal properties which fight against the causes of dandruff.

Here's a method of olive oil application to try:

You'll need:

- ½ cup of olive oil
- 5 drops of essential oil of choice (I use lavender)
- 1 plastic bag or shower cap

1. Pour olive oil in a jar with the oil and shake well. Let sit for 12 hours in cool, dark place and shake again before use
2. Wet the hair and scalp and take 1 tbsp. of the oil in the palm of your hand and using fingertips, gently massage into scalp using a circular motion.
3. Place bag or shower cap over hair for at least 1 hour before shampooing

What else works?

Lemon juice can be an excellent way to heal the scalp and treat dandruff. The acidity level of the lemon helps to balance the scalps pH level which in turn helps to keep dandruff at bay. Relief can be achieved by massaging 2 tbsp. of lemon juice into the scalp and rinsing with water. To maximize the results, try mixing the lemon juice with apple cider vinegar. The acetic acid helps to kill the fungus that causes dandruff.

How to apply remedy:

- Mix 4 tbsp. of ACV with 2 tbsp. of fresh lemon juice
- Apply all over scalp using fingers or cotton ball
  Repeat daily until dandruff disappears.

16-Migraine Headaches

A migraine is best described as a recurrent, throbbing headache usually on one side of the head and frequently accompanied by extreme sensitivity to light and sound. A migraine can also cause more distressing symptoms such as nausea, vomiting, and visual disturbances (aura).

If you've ever suffered with a migraine, you know how painfully debilitating it can be. This is because migraines are said to involve neurological as well as vascular changes in the brain during an attack. For sufferers, there seems to be a genetic component that is responsible for the reduced threshold for pain including the hypersensitivity to stimuli. This leads to increased migraine pain caused by the inflammation in the blood vessels surrounding the brain.

Chronic stress may be one of the most common causes of migraines and other headaches as well. Because of this, many alternative treatments aim at reducing stress such as relaxation and biofeedback and are highly effective for many migraine sufferers. In addition, other methods for treatment include acupuncture, herbs, and massage all of which provide varying levels of helpfulness.

Let's look at some relief options:

Essential Oils-*Lavender*, *peppermint*, and *basil* to be specific. These are all inexpensive and simple to use. Not to mention, they work great for migraine relief. Depending on your preference of oil (my personal favorite is peppermint), mix a few drops in 2 cups of boiling water. This can be used to breathe in the vapors with a towel over your head to help maximize the effect. In addition you can also apply the oil to the forehead and temples (dilute the peppermint oil prior to doing this). This remedy can be used 3 or more times per day to achieve relief.

Flaxseeds. Since migraines are essentially caused by inflammation, eating foods rich in Omega-3s can be helpful. Flaxseeds are rich in Omega-3s and can be enjoyed in several ways:

- Flaxseed oil-can be drizzled on salad or eaten by the spoon (refer to directions on bottle)
- Whole and ground flaxseeds can be added to smoothies and juices and sprinkled on cereal
- Ground flaxseeds can be added to bread mixture or soups

Last one:

Vicks Vaporub. In addition to being an excellent cough suppression, Vicks Vaporub is a wonderful cheap, home remedy for migraine headaches. Rub some Vicks onto the temples and forehead and then breathe in vapors. This can be repeated until the headache is gone!

17-Breast Cancer

This awful disease is responsible for the death of millions of women (and men) around the world yearly. It has caused so much paranoia and fear that many are opting for extreme precautionary measures such as mastectomies. This is an unfortunate fate that many are choosing for themselves regardless of the risks involved.

Because many people are unaware of the natural cures that exist, many are turning to their doctors and choosing harmful chemotherapy and radiation treatments. The problem with this is that these treatments actually promote more cancer in the long term as they destroy healthy cells and weaken the immune system further.

So where should a woman turn? They cannot count on their doctor to give them facts on natural treatments simply because their doctor does not know. Surely the pharmaceutical companies aren't planning on spilling the beans and risking billions of dollars' worth of medical treatments, no way.

Alternative treatments aren't only safer, but also backed up by several strong scientific literature. Let's begin looking at a few of them:

Vitamin D. This is only one of the several natural cures for breast cancer that have been said to work. It helps the body absorb calcium which is essential for maintaining bone health. In addition, Vitamin D helps to ensure that the immune system as well as the nervous system are healthy and functioning correctly.

Research suggests that Vitamin D may be effective at preventing breast cancer cells from forming. The best source of Vitamin D is the sun. This is why women and men are recommended to sunbathe for at least 30 minutes a day in order for their body to begin manufacturing the vitamin.

Here are some additional sources of Vitamin D to consider:

- Cod liver oil which is also rich in Vitamin D3, should be taken along with an additional vitamin D3 supplement.
- Salmon
- Herring
- Catfish
- Oysters
- Sardines
- Mackerel

What else can help cure breast cancer?

Baking Soda. Yes, we mention baking soda AGAIN. Simply because many swear by it for curing a wide variety of ailments including breast cancer. Best of all, it's cheap, and likely to be in your cabinet right now...go and get it!

Here's how to take it:

- 1 tsp. baking soda
- 2 tsp. grade B maple syrup or black strap molasses

Mix these two ingredients together on a spoon and take first thing in the morning. Make sure to stay hydrated by downing 1 full glass of water with this remedy. This can be continued for 4 weeks before resting. After resting for another 4 weeks, the protocol can be repeated.

Here's the final cure we'll look at:

Green Tea. We had mentioned Green Tea as a powerful remedy for diabetes. Did you know it is believed to be an effective treatment for breast cancer as well? No? Well now you know.

But what makes it great? Besides the fact that it contains extremely high levels of antioxidants known for neutralizing free radicals in the body, it also contains vitamin C and E. Also, natural chemicals contained in green tea not only prevent certain cancers from forming, they have even shown to reverse tumor growth. These remarkable benefits make green tea natures "wonder drug". Best of all, it's safe to drink every day!

18-Ovarian Cysts

Ovarian cysts are fluid-filled sacs within the ovaries that usually form during ovulation and dissolve after menstruation. They are extremely common in women of childbearing age and normally do not present any symptoms.

There are different types of ovarian cysts and most of them occur normally during the menstrual cycle making them functional. These types are normally benign and usually appear without any particular reason. There are however more serious types known as pathological cysts which can be either benign or cancerous.

Often times, women are not even aware that they have an ovarian cyst since they usually do not produce symptoms. However, in some cases, they can cause problems such as abdominal bloating, painful intercourse, menstrual irregularities, lower back and thigh pain, pressure in the rectum or bladder, nausea, and vomiting. More serious cases of ovarian cysts can even lead to infertility.

Depending on the type and size of the cyst, Doctor's may recommend the use of birth control pills or surgery to remove the ovaries and uterus. Although there are severe cases that may require these measures, the vast majority of cysts are functional and should only be addressed if they are presenting bothersome symptoms.

Ovarian cysts normally disappear on their own within a few short months. However, there are many natural remedies that can help relieve symptoms and even shrink the size of the cysts. Let's take a look:

Beetroot juice is an excellent ovarian cyst remedy that many people have had huge success with. Beetroot contains betacyanin which is a compound that helps boost the liver's ability to flush toxins out of the body. In addition, beetroot is naturally alkaline which can help decrease acidity in the body and since disease cannot survive in an alkaline environment, your body will be able to heal itself.

Recipe to try

- 1 cup of freshly extracted beetroot juice
- 1 tbsp. aloe vera gel
- 1 tbsp. blackstrap molasses

Drink this once daily prior to eating breakfast and repeat until your symptoms have reduced.

Apple Cider Vinegar. Ok, no brainer right? This miracle substance can cure just about anything what makes this disease any different?

Since a potassium deficiency can contribute to the formation of ovarian cysts, it's important to get enough of this mineral in your diet. Because ACV contains high levels of potassium it can help to shrink and virtually dissolve ovarian cysts when consumed regularly. In addition, it can help control blood sugars which prevents the release of excess insulin by the pancreas. High levels of insulin can lead to other issues such as elevated testosterone which is the main source of irregular menstrual cycles, increase in body hair and acne in women.

How to take

What you'll need:

- 1 tbsp. ACV
- 1 glass water
- 1 tbsp. blackstrap molasses

Mix ingredients together and drink twice daily until cysts have cleared up. For best results, avoid taking on an empty stomach to avoid digestive issues.

Finally...

Castor Oil Pack. This remedy goes back many centuries as a powerful way to draw toxins out of the body by stimulating the circulatory and lymphatic system. What's more, when placed on the lower abdomen, it can help circulate fresh nutrient-rich blood to reach the ovaries and help reduce or dissolve the cyst. This method can be very effective but its use is not recommended during menstruation.

How to use

1. Start by pouring about 2 tbsp. of castor oil onto a large piece of flannel cloth making sure to soak the entire cloth.
2. Place saturated cloth onto the abdomen area and secure it with plastic wrap.
3. Then, lay back and place a towel on top of the abdomen along with a hot water bottle (over the towel).
4. Leave on for 30-60 minutes and then remove and wash area.
5. This process can be repeated a couple of times a week for a duration lasting at least 2 months.

19-Brittle Nails

Everyone experiences brittle nails from time-to-time as they can be caused by numerous factors such as prolonged water exposure, aging, and through the long-term use of nail polish.

Weak, brittle nails chip fairly easily and many people describe them as cosmetically unappealing. Although the causes of brittle nails is normally benign, they can be caused by various diseases such as issues with the thyroid or lungs, psoriasis, alopecia areata, infections, and disorders of the endocrine system.

Other more common causes include dehydration, chemical exposure and nutritional deficiencies. Many times, a true cause cannot be pinpointed or could be due to multiple factors including the ones listed.

Nails that split or crack easily can cause some discomfort especially when the skin below the nail becomes exposed. When brittle nails are caused by nutritional deficiencies or an underlying medical problem, proper measures need to be taken to treat the condition first in order to experience long-term relief. There are however many natural home remedies that can help strengthen the nails regardless of the cause.

Let's take a look:

Sea Salt. This remedy is one that I hold dear to me as it has done wonders for my nails. Sea salt contains natural minerals that can help heal and strengthen brittle nails while adding some natural shine. In addition, it has an exfoliating effect which can help add softness to your cuticles.

How to use:

1. Mix 2 tbsp. sea salt in a small bowl of warm water.
2. Add two drops of essential oils of your choice (my favorite for this are frankincense and lemon).
3. Soak nails in the solution for up to 20 minutes.
4. Rinse off, and pat dry applying lotion shortly after.
5. This remedy is safe and can be repeated 3 times per week until positive results are achieved.

Let's look at the second remedy:

Lemon Juice can help in fortifying damaged nails and remove yellow stains on the nail surface leftover from nail polish. Olive oil can help enhance this remedy by providing moisture deep within the cuticles helping to strengthen nails. Mix the two together for optimal results.

Simply start by mixing 3 tbsp. olive oil and 1 tbsp. lemon juice in a small bowl. Heat the mixture just slightly and begin massaging into fingertips/nails. Leave on for 15 minutes and wash off. You should notice a significant difference after just a couple of treatments.

Tea Tree Oil. This was always my favorite go-to for various skin conditions such as acne due to its strong antiseptic properties. It is also useful for treating brittle nails especially when they are caused by fungal infections. In addition, it helps to treat discolored nails as well. This remedy is very simple to use and should be done daily until positive results have been achieved.

1. Begin by mixing ½ tsp. of olive oil or vitamin E oil with a few drops of the tea tree oil.
2. Rub mixture on nails while massaging for a few minutes.
3. Leave on for 20 minutes covering with plastic gloves to maximize the amount of penetration.
4. Rinse, pat dry, and follow up with lotion.

20-Irritable Bowel Syndrome (IBS)

According to the National Foundation for Functional Gastrointestinal Disorders, Irritable Bowel Syndrome (IBS) Affects between 25-45 million Americans per year with the vast majority of sufferers being women. Although the exact causes aren't known, disturbances within the nervous system, brain, and gut are thought to be linked to the disorder.

Experts have long believed that stress is the main culprit for IBS. However, it's less likely that stress actually causes IBS but rather can worsen or even trigger symptoms. This is due to the connection between the brain and gut. The underlying cause is often related to a poor-functioning digestive system which is worsened by a negative psychological state.

Unfortunately, millions of people suffer terribly and needlessly with this disorder and report a significantly diminished quality of life because of it. It's also important to note that IBS symptoms can mimic other more serious conditions. Because of this, it's important to have symptoms evaluated by a specialist prior to seeking treatments. Common IBS symptoms include:

- Abdominal pain and bloating
- Gas
- Constipation or diarrhea
- Nausea
- Fatigue
- Mucus in stool or when wiping
- Frequent urges to have a bowel movement

Standard medical treatments include anti-depressants, and anti-spasmodic drugs which do not address the underlying problems but rather treat the symptoms only. In the long run, these types of treatments can wreak havoc on gut by suppressing good bacteria causing, you guessed it, more intense symptoms.

Let's break this nasty cycle by looking at some natural remedies:

Peppermint oil. Peppermint is highly effective in treating IBS symptoms such as cramping, diarrhea, and bloating due to its menthol content. This has an antispasmodic effect within the digestive tract and can help food pass more easily through the stomach.

How to take:

- Add 4 drops of peppermint oil to 1/3 cup of warm water.

- Consume up to 4 times daily and continue until condition is improved.
- Peppermint tea can be also be used in the same frequency.

Let's see what else:

Yogurt containing live cultures has been known to reduce symptoms such as diarrhea in IBS sufferers. The friendly probiotic bacteria help to line the intestines creating a protective barrier that in turn flushes out toxins from the system. 3-4 servings of yogurt a day is best for maximum results and can be eaten by itself or added to smoothies. Try and limit sugar while doing this as sugar can have a reverse impact as bad bacteria within the gut will feed on it and multiply.

Final remedy:

Cabbage juice. Yuck! I know! But stay with me here, it isn't as bad as it sounds. Raw cabbage contains sulfur and chlorine which cleanses the stomach including the mucus membranes and intestines. It also has a laxative effect which can help soften bowels and heal any constipation symptoms in IBS sufferers. Not to mention, it helps keep the body hydrated which is the key to optimal overall health.

Instructions on how to take:

- Cut a head of cabbage into tiny pieces.
- Run through a juicer or blender to make juice.
  Drink about a half of a cup up to 4 times per daily to help maximize results.

Conclusion:

I am so glad you took the time out of your day to read through these powerful home remedies! Many of them have been used for centuries and are proven to help treat some of the most stubborn health conditions. I myself have used many of them and know others who have utilized them as well with successful results!

Remember if you're already taking medication for any of these conditions, make sure to consult your physician about these remedies in order to make sure there are no drug interactions. It's important that you NEVER abruptly stop taking any medications prior to talking to your doctor.

Since natural remedies can take longer to work than traditional medicine, it's important to stay persistent towards your health goals and remain patient in the process. Although pharmaceutical drugs can get rid of symptoms fairly quickly, they hardly treat the underlying cause. The results of going the natural route, can be far more drastic and effective as they work to treat underlying problems rather than just masking the symptoms.

I wish you great health, happiness, and prosperity!

CPSIA information can be obtained
at www.ICGtesting.com
Printed in the USA
LVHW011037150521
687531LV00015B/965